Medicine and Morality

Medicine and Morality

Crises in the History of a Profession

HELEN KANG

UBCPress · Vancouver · Toronto

28 27 26 25 24 23 22 21 20 19   5 4 3 2 1

Printed in Canada on FSC-certified ancient-forest-free paper (100% post-consumer recycled) that is processed chlorine-and acid-free.

Library and Archives Canada Cataloguing in Publication

Title: Medicine and morality : crises in the history of a profession / Helen Kang.
Names: Kang, Helen, author.
Description: Includes bibliographical references and index.
Identifiers: Canadiana (print) 20190163852 | Canadiana (ebook) 20190163860 |
    ISBN 9780774862127 (hardcover) | ISBN 9780774862134 (softcover) |
    ISBN 9780774862141 (PDF) | ISBN 9780774862158 (EPUB) |
    ISBN 9780774862165 (Kindle)
Subjects: LCSH: Medical ethics—Canada. | LCSH: Physicians—Professional ethics—
    Canada. | LCSH: Medical ethics—Canada—History. | LCSH: Physicians—
    Professional ethics—Canada—History. | LCSH: Conflict of interests—Canada.
Classification: LCC R724 .K36 2019 | DDC 174.20971—dc23

Canadä

UBC Press gratefully acknowledges the financial support for our publishing program of the Government of Canada (through the Canada Book Fund), the Canada Council for the Arts, and the British Columbia Arts Council.

This book has been published with the help of a grant from the Canadian Federation for the Humanities and Social Sciences, through the Awards to Scholarly Publications Program, using funds provided by the Social Sciences and Humanities Research Council of Canada.

Printed and bound in Canada by Friesens
Set in Myriad and Sabon by Apex CoVantage, LLC
Copy editor: Barbara Tessman
Proofreader: Alison Strobel
Indexer: Stephen Ullstrom
Cover designer: Will Brown

UBC Press
The University of British Columbia
2029 West Mall
Vancouver, BC V6T 1Z2
www.ubcpress.ca

For my parents, Sean and Kathy

Contents

Acknowledgments

This book has been published with the help of a grant from the Federation for the Humanities and Social Sciences, through the Awards to Scholarly Publications Program, using funds provided by the Social Sciences and Humanities Research Council of Canada. The original research was funded by the Social Science and Humanities Research Council Doctoral Fellowship.

This book was borne out of the help of many individuals. My gratitude goes to the following:

The editors at UBC Press, especially Darcy Cullen for believing in the possibility of this book at the proposal stage and James MacNevin for seeing me through the completion of the book, including the final peer review and approval by the UBC Press board.

The reviewers, for their insightful feedback and supportive comments that helped to morph what was an academic exercise into a true book.

Professor Cindy Patton, my doctoral senior supervisor, mentor, and friend. She nurtured me as a scholar and taught me to use my research skills for forces of good.

My committee members, Professors Dany Lacombe and Zoë Druick, as well as examiners Professors Nancy Tomes and Lara Campbell, for their thoughtful and engaged reading of the original research.

Jane Jones, for her gentle but firm coaching, which gave me the extra push I needed to finish the book.

M.T. O'Shaughnessy for offering me his critical insights and challenging my thinking about pertinent political and cultural issues in health, at a time when such spaces of reflection were not readily available to me.

Natasha Patterson, Joy Walcott-Francis, and Ayaka Yoshimizu – wonderful scholars and friends – as well as friends and colleagues I met through the Self-Employed PhD online community. Their creativity and commitment to intellectual work after their degree programs inspired me to write this book.

All the medical doctors I have worked with over the years, whose dedication to their patients, care, and the health care system remind me to be both compassionate and critical when engaging in critique of medicine.

My parents and my sister, who patiently saw me through my doctoral degree and gently encouraged me to finish the book.

My best friends and soul sisters, Shoshana Magnet and Shanta Varma. There are no words that adequately describe my love for these two amazing people who support me and challenge me to be the best person I can be in all aspects of life, including as a writer and thinker.

Last but not least, my partner in crime and in life, Dietrich Bassewitz, who has stood by my side through thick and thin and never ceased to be loving and encouraging, even during my many phases of self-discovery.

Medicine and Morality

Introduction

In recent years, critics of biomedicine, including physicians and medical researchers, have become increasingly concerned about the problem of conflict of interest in that field. "Conflict of interest," in this context, has been broadly defined as the damaging impact of economic, political, and personal interests on what should be the "pure" scientific and moral imperative of medicine to be objective and to do no harm. Those with concerns about conflict of interest have focused mostly on interactions between medical practitioners, researchers, and the multimillion-dollar pharmaceutical industry. The impact of Big Pharma on medical knowledge and practices has been well documented, including the influence of "detailing" by drug sales-representatives on the prescribing practices of clinicians, the potential bias-inducing impact of privatization and drug industry funding on biomedical research, and the close relationship between the industry and medical schools.[1]

The role of drug industry forces in medicine is an important issue with wide-reaching social, political, and ethical implications for public health, patient care, and scientific knowledge. However, current discussions about medical conflict of interest offer only a limited view of the types of such conflicts that exist, and have existed, in medicine, how they arise, and how medical professionals conceptualize and respond to them in the pursuit of health and the protection of patients from harm. Current discussions treat conflict of interest as a contemporary phenomenon, coinciding with the emergence of the Big Pharma in the mid-twentieth century, rather than placing it in a historical context. While serious, drug industry influence accounts for only a fraction of the types of conflict of interest that doctors and the medical profession have faced, and continue to face. In the late nineteenth and early twentieth centuries, doctors lobbied various levels of government for laws that would grant the medical profession autonomy and self-regulating powers, as a way to eradicate other health practitioners who threatened the medical profession's dominance in the medical market. In mid-twentieth century, when the Saskatchewan government led by Thomas C. ("Tommy") Douglas moved to institute a publicly funded health insurance plan, the Saskatchewan Medical Association and the College of Physicians and Surgeons of Saskatchewan vehemently opposed the proposal, organizing a doctors' strike in 1962 that drew considerable public criticism, including in the national press. In these moments, the professional interests of medicine stood at odds with those of the state, other professional groups, and even the public.

Medical professionals are expected to act in the interests of patients and the health of the public – that is, of someone other than themselves. If doctors are involved in research as clinician-researchers, they are expected to act in the interest of scientific progress, the pursuit of knowledge, and the common good – that is, for something beyond their own personal interests. At the same time that they are held to these moral and scientific standards, doctors are rewarded individually and collectively for acting in the interests of others. They often have high incomes, have respectable careers as professionals, and are recognized by the state, the media, and the legal system as experts whose statements about health and illness have tremendous value and credibility. In medicine, there is a tension between the necessary evils of depending on the market economy and state politics for sources of monies and legislative support, and medicine's genuine investment in the pursuit of moral integrity, scientific innovation, objectivity, and neutrality. In other words, for doctors, being medical professionals is a moral paradox.

In this book, I move beyond current considerations around conflict of interest to consider more broadly the ways in which moral and scientific norms in medicine have emerged and evolved over time. Standards with regard to what is moral and what is scientific are not fixed or abstract; rather, they are historically constituted in relation to social, political, economic, and cultural forces. In the following chapters, I focus on historical moments when patients, journalists, and politicians, all of whom are invested in how medicine is done, questioned doctors' moral and scientific authority. In these moments of moral crisis, the medical profession responded by re-evaluating, rearticulating, and even reshaping what it meant for doctors to act with moral and scientific integrity, doing so in ways that legitimated particular practices with respect to their relationship to the public, the media, and politics, with wide-reaching implications. As I will show, medical professionals have pursued moral and scientific integrity in direct relation to, rather than in spite of, conflict of interest. As they have butted up against other stakeholders in health and medicine, they have shaped what ought and ought not to be done in the name of patient care, public health, and scientific objectivity.

Science, Morality, and Medicine

Medicine straddles multiple domains: it is a science that produces knowledge about the human body; it is an art that bridges the biological and social dimensions of life; it is a moral enterprise that deals in the intimacies of life and death. The medical doctor sits at the intersection of these concerns, grappling with the daily pursuit of benevolence, non-maleficence, scientific objectivity, accountability, respectability, and all the other ideals of the medical professional. Medicine and its practitioners are popular subjects in various disciplines, including history, sociology, anthropology, cultural studies, and the social study of science. Some writers take medicine's own claims to be scientific and morally upright at face value as unquestionable justification for the authority and credibility of the profession. Others are skeptical of the medical profession's moral and scientific claims, treating these claims as the tools of persuasion through which the profession exerts its political power and social dominance. Still others take a more discursive approach, examining practices and language through which medicine articulates and shapes its ideas of "science" and "morality" and, by extension, examining what it means to enact scientificness and moral integrity in the clinical, scientific, and political pursuits of medicine.

Noble Origins and the Myth of Progress

Ideas related to "science" and "morality" figure centrally in the history of the medical profession, particularly in the profession's own narrative about its origins. The earliest texts about doctors in Canada were written by doctors themselves.[2] These physician-historians portrayed the medical profession as a noble group of "medical men," as they called themselves, deserving the authority to oversee all matters surrounding health and disease. These historical texts often served political purposes for the emerging profession, as doctors struggled to gain professional legitimacy, both in the eyes of governments and among the physicians whom it claimed to represent.

One of the first publications about the medical profession in Canada is William Canniff's *The Medical Profession in Upper Canada, 1783–1850*, published in 1894. The text is decidedly conservative and pro-British, emphasizing the legislative triumphs by British physicians and surgeons to raise the status of their profession over and above that of their competitors, such as homeopaths and other "quacks." During a time when French-British tensions in Canada were high, a primarily British-centric historical account would have served as a way for English-speaking medical men to establish a sense of their common history.[3] H.E. MacDermot's *History of the Canadian Medical Association, 1867–1921*, which was first published in 1935 by the Canadian Medical Association, echoes Canniff's narrative structure. He documents the trials facing medical men during the late nineteenth century as they nobly struggled against what he describes as rampant quackery and ignorance among the masses. In Canniff's and MacDermot's accounts, medical men are already united as a profession with a common set of goals and ideals, including the dominance of Anglo medical doctors and of the British system of professionalization. Both authors claim that scientific innovation and progress in medicine led to the (rightful) dominance and credibility of medical men over other practitioners. Their explicitly self-aggrandizing tone points to a sense of urgency among medical men to legitimize their professional status and respectability.

Their line of argument appears in later historical texts as well.[4] Often, these texts subscribe to the progress myth that better science led to better medicine. These authors claim that the social and political constraints faced by the medical profession in the nineteenth century were resolved by the miracle of scientific innovation and progress in the twentieth century. For example, Colin D. Howell writes that doctors in the nineteenth century could not agree on what counted as legitimate medical knowledge, nor were they substantially different from untrained practitioners in their therapeutic approaches and rates of clinical success. However, he concludes that doctors rose to their eventual expert status by accepting "popular notions of the value of science and responsible social management,"[5] as though "the value of science" and "responsible social management" were concepts that already existed during this time and that doctors simply needed to accept.

Critical writings and historical analyses of medicine by non-physicians from the 1980s onwards provide a more nuanced way of understanding the relationship between morality, science, and medical knowledge and practices. Academic historians in Canada began to problematize the assumption in earlier literature that medical men had always been united as a homogeneous group, pointing to the scientific, political, and social conflicts that shaped medical practice, in particular the medical profession's struggles to claim moral and scientific superiority over other healing professions.[6]

S.E.D. Shortt argues in a 1983 essay that the trend in the historiography of medicine to unproblematically link "the professionalization of medicine in a causal fashion to a growth in scientific knowledge requires substantial modification."[7] He then describes the ways in which science as a form of "polite knowledge" was a tool used by Victorian middle-class physicians in the Americas to forge a group identity, one that was distinct from upper-class medical men.[8] In doing so, Shortt situates scientific discourse, class struggles, morality, and legitimacy in the same relational space. In a similar vein, Paul Underhill's analysis of the medical reform movement in Britain demonstrates that the social and political conflicts among British medical men overlapped with disputes about the very nature of medicine as a body of knowledge and practice.[9] In her book *History of Medicine: A Scandalously Short Introduction*, Jaclyn

Duffin also situates the creation of the medical profession in Canada in the context of the social and political roles of physicians in the construction of knowledge about the human body and about disease.[10] Standards of scientificness and the pursuit of moral integrity in medicine are not separate from doctors' socio-political struggles. Medicine's discourses, practices, and actions around "morality" and "science" are part and parcel of professional medicine's pursuit of legitimacy and authority.

Medical Dominance and Medicine as Culture

Ideas about medicine's authority and power form a central concern in a large body of sociological literature. Rooted in structuralist approaches and political economy traditions, these analyses focus on the concept of "medical dominance," or the medical profession's power "over the content of their own work (characterised as autonomy) and its power over the work of other health care occupations (authority) as institutionalised experts in all matters relating to health in the wider society (sovereignty)."[11] These texts trace the emergence of medical dominance to the early days of the profession in the nineteenth century, during which medical doctors battled other healing practitioners – and won. The lines of inquiry tend to revolve around whether or not the medical profession has or had dominance and the degree to which this dominance may have been eroded in the health care workplace, in policy making and legislation, and in relation to other health professions and patients.[12]

In the structural analyses of doctors as a profession, ethics/morality and science are either moot points or vehicles for the profession's more pressing concerns in establishing and maintaining structural power. In this literature, science is taken up primarily in the form of "medicalization," or the adoption of formerly non-medical issues into the realm of medical knowledge and expertise, a process that serves to reinforce the authority and dominance of professional medicine.[13] The pursuit of dominance is so central to this body of work that Ronald Hamowy goes as far as to state that "it is foolish to suppose that their occupation exalts them above using the means at their disposal to act in their own private interests," a view he diametrically contrasts with the medical profession's own assertion that "its dedication is the public's interest" and "that [doctors] have never sought legislation or acted for selfish ends."[14]

Another type of sociological literature, which emerges from symbolic traditions, treats the profession as a type of culture and examines science and morality in relation to cultural norms and identity formation in medicine. Drawing on anthropological approaches and often presented through ethnographic studies, these works emphasize the ways in which doctors at various stages in their careers – including as medical students[15] and junior doctors[16] – and in various working contexts – such as emergency wards[17] – conduct themselves in relation to expectations from patients, other doctors, and managers. These works emphasize behaviours of and perceptions held by doctors and medical students in relation to the situations and conflicts in which they find themselves[18] in the context of a hierarchized professional culture.[19] Some of these works take up Pierre Bourdieu's concept of "habitus" in order to describe a "medical habitus," which is cast primarily as doctors' identity[20] and embodied clinical practices,[21] and is seen as being shaped via encounters with professional and health care institutions. In these works, the structures of professional culture, among which are scientific practices and moral standards, largely shape the professional identities and embodied practices of doctors.

David Armstrong takes a symbolic approach in his analyses of moral and ethical issues in medicine. In one essay, he finds that doctors observe professional etiquette as a communicative strategy that helps them mediate conflicting opinions around prescribing treatments without compromising clinical autonomy, which he defines as the ability of a doctor to make clinical decisions free from intervention by others, including other doctors.[22] Armstrong has also analyzed the significance of early medical professional codes of ethics (from the nineteenth century onward) in terms of the socio-political concerns of the profession during various time periods.[23] For instance, he finds that nineteenth-century codes demonstrate a metaphoric parallel with the public health approaches at the time, which were concerned with monitoring the boundaries of the body – the public body, the individual body, and the professional body – to guard them from contaminants, including diseases and unfit doctors.

Armstrong's work shows how professional medicine's socio-political interest in authority and legitimacy – ensuring that doctors are seen as experts on all matters of health and illness – and individual physicians' struggle to practise medicine as they see fit interact with and manifest themselves in everyday practice, such as in clinical decision-making and codes of ethics. The ways in which doctors perceive themselves as autonomous experts and hold themselves to specific ethical norms are part of the daily culture of medicine, which in turn is inseparable from the profession's socio-political struggles. Medicine's moral and scientific claims are not only political strategies to gain authority and power but are also practices that shape the culture of medicine as lived by doctors, particularly when they relate to one another, their patients, and others who have a stake in how care and medicine is done.

Medicine as a Discursive Space

Language and representation are key features of any culture, including the culture of medicine. The ways in which the field of medicine as a whole articulates what it knows, how it knows what it knows, what it does, and why it does what it does offer a window into its understandings of the norms of science and morality in medicine. The study of medical discourse is largely considered to begin with the work of Michel Foucault, particularly his *Madness and Civilization* and *The Birth of the Clinic*,[24] both of which moved away from established narratives of scientific progress, discoveries, and innovations as well as investigation of origins and causes of medical theories and practices. Foucault emphasized patterns of discursive formation, such as the development of new objects and lexicons related to medical knowledge, to institutional networks, and to new ways of seeing and organizing what is knowable. His concept of the "medical gaze" was an alternative to medicalization[25] as a way to understand the power of physicians, which he saw as the capacity and the authority to draw on the entire discourse and institution of medicine when using their gaze and touch in clinical practice.

Foucault's work has inspired a vast range of writing that examines the discursive impact of medical techniques and knowledge, such as diagnostic strategies, clinical categories,[26] and visualizations of the body.[27] The interdisciplinary area of social studies of science and medicine combines influences from the sociology of knowledge, cultural studies, and the history of science and medicine to engage with scientific knowledge and practices as part of the social, cultural, and political lives of scientists and health professionals. By treating medicine as a discursive space that is susceptible to broader socio-political forces and systems of oppression, scholars have framed medicine as a political space in which the human body is imagined and worked on in order to produce docile bodies,[28] new regulatory regimes,[29] and new ways for medicine to know what it knows.[30] Feminist and critical race scholars emphasize that biomedical knowledge and practices continue to produce particularly gendered and racialized bodies and subjectivities, often in concert with other discourses such as those related to law, citizenship, sexuality, colonization, and religion.[31]

The works that draw on Foucault's approach have highlighted the ways in which medical thinking is heterogeneous and often inconsistent across time and disciplinary boundaries, thereby debunking assumptions about the immutability of scientific facts and truths.[32] Drawing on Foucault's work, science historians Lorraine Daston and Peter Galison argue that, historically in Western science, the standards of what constitutes an objective manner by which a scientist may observe and represent a phenomenon to other scientists were entwined with ideas around moral integrity and self-cultivation of the scientist – specifically, in scientists' ability to control the subjectivity of their gaze and follow the established procedures of observation at the time.[33] Scientific ways of seeing have thus always been inseparable from moral ways of being scientific.

In medicine, the interrelationship between science and morality is evident in the ways in which doctors present themselves to one another and to their patients. Lianne McTavish examines medical treatises written by male midwives in nineteenth-century France. These men deployed visual and textual practices of self-representation that helped them gain credibility during a time when women dominated midwifery. McTavish argues that male midwives often represented themselves as gender hybrids in order to downplay the sexual danger of their presence in the birthing chamber. At the same time, they highlighted their gendered privilege as men, who were considered to be more theoretically competent than women.[34] Working on a similar historical period, Robert Nye finds that scientists and medical men of Victorian England and modern Europe adopted the old duelling codes of aristocratic men as a socially appropriate way to resolve conflict between one another over scientific views.[35] He draws on the works of science historians Steven Shapin[36] and Mario Biagioli[37] on early modern scientists, for whom personal honour was closely associated with scientific credibility. McTavish and Nye demonstrate that doctors used moralized strategies around gender and class in order to gain credibility, and that these practices were also related to scientific standards and norms of the time.

The discursive relationship between morality and scientificness plays out in the clinic and medical research as well. Kathryn Montgomery[38] combines literary analysis of doctors in fictional narratives with ethnographic observations of medical students in order to examine the ways in which doctors come to think the way they do, particularly as they navigate the uncertainties and messiness of medical practice. She argues that clinical judgment is often based on non-scientific knowledge and practices[39] and asserts that the moral and the clinical are intertwined in the context of medical practice. By insisting that medicine is foremost a science, physicians can block empathetic relations with their patients, thereby de-emphasizing the moral basis for the therapeutic practice of medicine. The tension between the moral and the clinical is one of the foci of Lisa Keränen's *Scientific Characters: Rhetoric, Politics, and Trust in Breast Cancer Research*.[40] She explores a recent scandal in Canadian breast cancer research, where a prominent scientist in the field was found to have falsified data for decades. In her analysis of the ways in which the scientist was characterized, Keränen identifies tensions in the figure of the researcher-physician, who must be both a beneficent healer and a career-minded scientist. She links this tension to different norms of what a proper and moral physician-scientist must be.

Doctors negotiate moral and scientific standards through the ways in which they engage with others in the profession as well as those outside of it, particularly patients and the public, on whose behalf doctors are supposed to act. A close examination of the discursive practices through which they present themselves as moral and scientific subjects yields insight into what exactly is meant by "moral" and "scientific" and which practices and ideas are permissible within medicine in the name of these ideals – and which are not.

Understanding Scientific and Moral Norms in Context

French anthropologist Pierre Bourdieu argues that in most social spaces, such as the economic market, schools, politics, and the media, people compete with one another in the interest of themselves, their family networks, and other social groups to which they belong. However, in certain pockets of society, people display interests that go beyond the self, such as in the religious callings of priests, aesthetic visions of artists, and objective commitments of scientists. Altruism, selflessness, and the desire to pursue something – art, knowledge, and so on – for its own sake are some of the qualities that we as a culture associate with people from these social worlds. Bourdieu calls these social spaces "anti-economic universes"[41] because the logic by which they operate is opposite that of a conventional economy, with the latter characterized by competition, self-advancement, and barter/exchange of goods and services. He argues further that artists, priests, and scientists are personally rewarded for acting in the interest of something or someone other than themselves, an outcome that contradicts the selfless premise of their actions. For instance, scientists compete with one another for research funding, recognition, publication, and rewards, although they do so in the name of progress, the common good, and the pursuit of knowledge for the sake of knowledge. Scientists act in the interest of something other than themselves, but to do so they engage in self-interested acts: they act with what Bourdieu calls "invested disinterestedness." He does not dismiss invested disinterestedness as a lie or a delusion that masks supposedly truer and more selfish intentions, nor does he naively take disinterested claims at face value. Instead, he describes such disinterestedness as a genuine motivation, at the same time that it is socially strategic.

Similarly, we can see doctors' claims to be disinterested as a genuine belief that what they do is on behalf of someone, and in the interest of something, beyond themselves. At the same time, we can see these claims as socially, politically, and culturally strategic in maintaining doctors' authority and legitimacy as experts on matters of health and illness. The moral and scientific standards in medicine are determined by a system of rewards that cannot be explained solely by an economic model based on a self-interested and calculating subject, or by an ahistorical and apolitical view of morality in terms of altruism and pure selflessness. Indeed, for doctors and scientists alike, self-interested and disinterested actions – or economic and anti-economic practices – are not easily distinguishable. Without money for health care through private and/or public insurance systems, medical care is not possible in current health care models. Without money for research, whether it is privately sourced through industry or publicly acquired through government grants, life-saving medications and technologies would be severely limited. Recognition from other scientists and clinicians determines the value of scientific work, and the intellectual work of science relies on centuries of generating, testing, and refuting theories by generations of scientists, a process that engenders, and also benefits from, competition. As much as doctors and scientists may claim that their work is for the common good, they also struggle with hospital and university administrations and the state to ensure that they are paid satisfactorily for their services. According to Bourdieu, anti-economic universes implicitly, and necessarily, rely on economic forces. Moreover, this contradiction is held together by a genuine collective denial of this paradox.

Rather than focus on whether or not doctors' claims to be disinterested are valid, which is a valuable line of inquiry that I leave to other scholars and analysts, I examine in this book how the delicate contradiction between self-interestedness and disinterestedness is held together in medicine, particularly in moments where the contradiction becomes so obvious that the collective denial risks falling apart. These are crisis moments when the medical profession's claims to scientific and moral legitimacy have been put into question by doctors themselves, the public, the media, and politicians, to the point where the profession was compelled to re-examine its priorities, strategize about ways to regain credibility, and redefine what it meant to be a good doctor.

Science and morality are cultural concepts that shift across time and are defined through social, cultural, and political struggles. Thus, what are considered to be matters of science, morality, and ethics today may not have been thought of as such in other moments in history. Conversely, what were considered to be matters of scientific and moral importance in other historical moments may not be recognized as such today. Keeping this historical specificity in mind, throughout this book I avoid judging doctors' actions as moral or scientific according to current standards. Instead, I pay attention to the specific scientific and moral priorities for doctors during each crisis moment, the kinds of conflicting interests they faced in relation to these priorities, and how they struggled to restore their scientific and moral legitimacy, in the process generating new possibilities of what it meant to do medicine and to be a medical professional. To do so, I examine how doctors expressed their scientific and moral concerns in editorial content in medical journals. Written by (physician) editors of journals published for their colleagues, these editorials are non-scientific texts that contain thoughts and arguments about social, political, cultural, and professional issues that doctors face. The medical journals also publish letters by (physician) readers responding to editorial content. Together these sources serve as a window into how doctors at various times in history highlighted, discussed, and debated matters of scientific and moral importance.

In Chapter 1, I outline in greater detail the concept of medical disinterestedness, which is a map that will guide the reader through the remainder of the book. Drawing on Bourdieu's concept of invested disinterestedness, I develop an analytical framework that takes scientific and moral standards seriously as part of doctors' endeavours to strive for integrity in medicine, and that also accounts for the kinds of social, cultural, and political struggles that doctors faced in the pursuit of authority, expertise, and legitimacy. For Bourdieu, invested disinterestedness is a particular kind of moral disposition and moral order, which emerged in the nineteenth century in concurrence with the rise of the bourgeoisie and the dramatic reorganization of economic, political, and cultural capitals in Europe. By tracing the details of this concept across his works, I posit that medical disinterestedness helps us understand how doctors in Canada, as particular socio-political agents, have developed their scientific and moral ethos and modified it over time, in direct relation to the kinds of conflicts and struggles they faced.

Subsequent chapters examine three crisis moments in the history of the Canadian medical profession, during which doctors' claim to scientific and moral integrity were questioned by the public, the media, and the state. Chapter 2 takes place in the nineteenth century and examines the emergence of medical disinterestedness during a time when doctors in Canada struggled to come together as a cohesive group of professionals recognized by the public and the state as legitimate experts. Doctors at this time were entrepreneurs, competing with one another and with other non-medical practitioners, such as homeopaths, yet offering very few remedies to their patients that differentiated them from the "quacks," as doctors called these alternative practitioners. The ideal of a scientifically and morally upright doctor, who was a member of a respectable profession, was shaped in the image of the British gentleman, as a direct result of the ethnic, gender, and class conflicts among doctors in this period. At the same time that doctors came together under the banner of the (British) gentleman, they moved away from portraying themselves as self-serving businessmen, frustrated by competition and a lack of regulation by the state, to instead present themselves as moral and scientific agents who practised their craft for the well-being of their patients and the good of the public.

Despite doctors' claim to act in the interest of their patients and the public, they still expected to be paid for their services. The thorny issue of payment for disinterested acts became the heart of a major controversy in the history of Canadian medicine in 1962, which is the setting for Chapter 3. On 1 July of that year, the medical profession in Saskatchewan, with the support of the national medical association, staged a day-long strike in protest against a provincial government proposal to establish a tax-funded, state-administered health insurance system – what is now the cornerstone of the current Canadian health care system. Saskatchewan doctors were intensely criticized in the national media for acting selfishly to protect their lucrative incomes instead of responding to the financial needs of patients – the first time that the Canadian medical profession encountered such profound public distrust with respect to its integrity. As the Canadian medical profession struggled to mend its relationship with the public, doctors began to discuss the idea that they needed to conduct better public relations and media relations, practices they had previously associated with corporate advertising and war propaganda. Doctors came to argue that a close medicine-media relationship was a way for them to be more socially responsible, and thus for the medical profession to better fulfill its moral duties toward the public.

In Chapter 4, I examine how the close medicine-media relationship lay the ground for another controversy involving Canadian doctors, one in which the interests of journalism and the media conflicted with the scientific interests of medicine. In 2006, the senior editors of the *Canadian Medical Association Journal* (*CMAJ*) were fired by the journal owners, spurring an international outcry that editorial freedom had been violated. However, the significance of the event went beyond editorial freedom, with profound implications for medical publishing. The antagonistic relationship between the editors and the owners of the *CMAJ* was based on conflicting interests between the two parties about what the journal should contain. The editors wanted to engage in journalistic reporting as well as scientific publishing, thereby fulfilling medicine's social responsibility to engage in social and political issues. The owners wanted to avoid such engagement and argued that the journal should uphold "pure" science instead. In this discursive battle over what was moral, what was scientific, and which of the two was a higher priority for medical publishing, the economic forces of the media industry – that is, how to finance a publication – constantly loomed large as a factor that could jeopardize both concerns.

This book is not a history of the medical profession in Canada, nor is it a history of how medicine in Canada became more scientific and morally reliable as a profession. Rather, it is about claims. Specifically, it is about claims to moral integrity and credibility made by a particular group of people – medical doctors – during times when this credibility was brought into question. Notions of "science" and "morality" in medicine are constantly being rewritten and reimagined with every conflict and question, large and small, about the legitimacy and accountability of doctors. I invite the reader to go beyond the contemporary emphasis on the presence or absence of industry ties among doctors as the primary site of conflicts in medicine. Instead, I urge the reader to examine more broadly problems of ethics, social responsibility, professionalism, integrity, and objectivity that emerge when the interests of doctors conflict with those of the public, the media, politicians, and state bureaucrats, and with those of other doctors.

Toward a Theory of Medical Disinterestedness 1

The world of doctors is unique. Like scientists, artists, and religious fig-ures, whose goal is to act on behalf of something other than economic self-interest (for example, knowledge, beauty, creativity, innovation, faith, God), doctors' primary motivation is to act on behalf of others, with a focus on the health and well-being of their patients and the public in general. Medical ethics are founded on this notion of acting on behalf of others: to do good by others (benevolence), to do no harm to others (non-maleficence), and to stand up for others (advocacy). The success of individual doctors, and the medical profession as a whole, depends on how well they can act on behalf of others. The rewards of this success are promotions, higher income, prestige, and greater power and authority. Ironically, then, the rewards of selflessness are self-advancement.

To dismiss this contradiction as a lie or to naively accept medicine's claims to selflessness as altruism misses important nuances and ethical questions that emerge when this logic operates in situ. To understand this contradictory logic of the world of doctors and how it operates in prac-tice, we turn to Pierre Bourdieu's concept of invested disinterestedness. To conceptualize the fine nuances of invested disinterestedness, as both a motivation and a social norm, I begin with his foundational concepts of field, capital, and habitus and then examine some of his secondary concepts, such as symbolic capital, field autonomy, and double habitus.

Bourdieu's work on the scientific field in particular provides a framework for understanding the field of medicine, and so I use the terms "scientific field" and "medical field" interchangeably in this chapter.

The Game Is Not a Game

Bourdieu often uses the analogy of a game to explain how he sees the social world. The social game unfolds in a field. For Bourdieu, the "field" is a conceptual space where social struggles take place and where various social, political, economic, and cultural forces operate. The game is governed by rules, or forces, which define the stakes and which constrain the moves players are allowed to make. For any game to exist, there must also exist players who are invested in playing the game in the first place and who possess some capacity to make the moves that are required. This capacity of the players is what Bourdieu refers to as the "habitus," or the disposition that one develops through long immersion in a field and that one needs in order to play the game. The habitus includes tacit knowledge of how to play the game, the lens through which to see the world, and the internal sense of how to act in any given situation. All this is developed over time through socialization in social institutions, such as education, family, traditions, the state, and the media.

When people play a social game, they do so in the pursuit of certain stakes, or what Bourdieu calls "capital." Field, capital, and habitus are interlinked concepts that help us map a given social world at a given time. Bourdieu draws the term "capital" from Marx but uses it to encompass more than just economic capital: capital is any object, skill, or decree that is deemed to be of value at a given time in a given social space. In addition to economic capital, which is anything that is a measurement of wealth, there are cultural capital, educational capital, social capital, and symbolic capital. "Cultural capital" refers to a person's knowledge, know-how, and sensibility to recognize and appreciate certain cultural objects and activities that are deemed valuable within a field. It includes knowledge of books, cultural references, music, and art, and competency in languages and sport. An individual's family of origin and upbringing can affect that person's exposure to certain cultural objects and practices, through the availability of book or other media. Formal training in cultural practices, such as music lessons or language classes in one's mother tongue, can also affect an individual's cultural capital. "Educational capital" includes degrees, diplomas, and certifications that affect access to employment and, eventually, one's income and wealth. "Social capital" includes affective and supportive relations, such as family, friends, and acquaintances.[1] No form of capital has value in and of itself outside of the field in which it operates, because, to continue the game analogy, the stakes have no value outside of the game. Each species of capital can convert into another species – for example, educational capital can convert into economic capital – and the conversion rate changes according to changes in the field.

"Scientific capital" functions as a type of symbolic capital, according to Bourdieu. Among the various species of capital he addresses in his work, symbolic capital is the most elusive. He defines it as honour, prestige, status, titles, and family name, all of which are exclusively tied to an individual and cannot be transferred to another.[2] The concept first appears in Bourdieu's often-cited ethnographic analysis of the gift economy in the Algerian village of Kabylia.[3] He observes that the villagers always followed a gift with a counter-gift but allowed some time to lapse before offering the counter-gift. If a gift receiver were to offer the counter-gift too soon, it would be considered a grave insult to the original gift-giver because it would suggest that the gift exchange was actually barter. The social conventions of this society required everyone involved to explicitly and actively deny that the practice of gift giving was, in fact, an economic exchange.[4] At stake in this game of the gift was honour, both in the act of giving a gift and returning a counter-gift. For the gift giver, this honour implicitly functioned as credit – the gift receiver was symbolically indebted to the gift giver – but this fact was denied in order for this entire interchange to be thought of as a gift, not barter exchange. Bourdieu warns that to dismiss this denial as an illusion or a lie undermines an intricate practice that was central to the village's social fabric.

In addition to relying on collective denial, symbolic capital operates by an entirely opposite logic to that of economic capital, while at the same time relying on economic capital to function properly. Examining European history and cultures, Bourdieu argues that the professional and ruling classes strive to win public recognition that they are honourable and respectable as a result of having certain forms of economic and cultural capital (e.g., their educational credentials). These groups mobilize their symbolic capital in order to influence and shape the perception of the world and the structures of the field. For example, medical doctors and lawyers may convert the reputation and respectability of their professions in order to run as political candidates or seek positions in policy making, and once in these positions they enact laws and policies that affect large groups of people.[5] People who possess symbolic capital command recognition without having to exert force and can influence the rules of the game simply by claiming to speak on behalf of those who provided them with recognition in the first place. Drawing on Max Weber's concept of charisma, Bourdieu argues that the state can engender submission, without having to explicitly demand it, by relying on feelings of honour, recognition, and credit, all of which tend to obscure the economic and physical forces (e.g., monopoly, the military) through which the state acquired its symbolic capital in the first place.[6] Thus, elected officials can claim to speak on behalf of their constituents, when in fact it was members of their own socio-economic class – those who possessed the economic, cultural, and political capital – who created the system of governance in the first place.

When Bourdieu states that symbolic capital is "nothing more than economic or cultural capital when it is known and recognized,"[7] he demystifies the power of those in dominant positions. However, his empirical work also tells us that symbolic capital works only when it is unknown and unrecognized (or, alternatively when players refuse to know or recognize) it. The players who are invested in the game must collectively deny the fact that there is an economy at work; instead, they must pursue honour, whether it is through the supposedly selfless act of gift giving or the supposedly selfless act of being a public servant. Invested disinterestedness is this collective denial of the game as a game and the collective investment in honour. The logic of invested disinterestedness allows an exchange of goods to be called a gift and someone who mobilizes wealth and credentials to win a political seat a servant of the public.

In most social worlds, players knowingly engage in competition and struggle for capital. There is a shared understanding among all the players that, for example, individuals are graded and evaluated in schools vis-à-vis others in class in order to then be granted degrees, diplomas, and opportunities that will eventually place them on different rungs of the economic hierarchy. In the scientific field, which Bourdieu calls a type of "anti-economic universe," players collectively deny that a game is taking place. Scientific capital is primarily prestige and honour – for example, to be cited by others and for one's name to be known in one's intellectual circles as someone of influence. The accepted objective of the game is not to better one's own position in the field but to contribute to the collective work toward something beyond the self – the common good and the pursuit of knowledge for its own sake. The denial lies in the unspoken truth that, by successfully acting in the interest of something or someone else, one betters one's own position. The game is not a game.

Invested Disinterestedness

Invested disinterestedness is an empirical concept that appears sporadically across Bourdieu's ethnographic works. The concept, as I use it in this book with regard to the moral and scientific norms in medicine, emerged in the historical context of major cultural, social, economic, and political changes that took place in Europe in the late eighteenth and nineteenth centuries – namely, the decline of the aristocracy and the monarchy, and the rise of the bourgeoisie, which included scientists and doctors. Medical disinterestedness is inseparable from the rise of the bourgeoisie, a new social class that developed its own unique habitus, including a moral ethos, in relation to new political and economic structures in Europe that would then spread to its former colonies.

In Bourdieu's field theory, the rules of the game not only dictate which forms of capital are at stake but also determine the rates of conversion between different species of capital.[8] Prior to the fall of the aristocracy and the monarchy in Europe, having a royal or aristocratic family name translated into the ability to rule. No other class had the means of possessing the political capital to rule, since the only way one could govern was by having royal or aristocratic lineage. In the nineteenth century, most major European monarchies declined and aristocracies were severely pruned. In Bourdieu-speak, this meant that the conversion link between symbolic capital in the form of royal or aristocratic lineage and political capital was broken and that, with the redistribution of wealth that ensued, the game of political rule became open to new stakes, new rules, and new players. Groups that had once been barred from the game – those outside the monarchy and aristocracy – could potentially rewrite the rules to make their own sets of assets, skills, and know-how the dominant forms of capital.

An important new player during this period was the bourgeoisie, which emerged as a new social class. This new kid on the block sought to set itself apart from the other existing social classes – the working class, the aristocracy, and the monarchy. Bourdieu argues that, while the aristocracy of the Old World relied on spectacles of consumption in order to enact its dominance over the peasants, the bourgeoisie enacted its position in the class struggle through restraint. However, this restraint was possible only within a condition of affluence. Possessing wealth allowed the bourgeoisie the luxury of not concerning itself with everyday necessities, such as making a living, putting food on the table, and paying the bills, and thus being able to focus on ease, leisure, and selective luxury.[9] Bourdieu finds that the bourgeoisie became invested in things outside of basic life necessities as a way to set itself apart from the working class, whose time and activities are more closely aligned with securing life's necessities. At the same time, the bourgeoisie could distinguish itself from the aristocracy and the former monarchy by demonstrating restraint when it came to enjoying luxuries.

In addition to being traits of the bourgeoisie's class identity, leisure and restraint translated into the bourgeoisie's political ethos – to be concerned with the universal, beyond day-to-day survival, and to act in the interest of something and someone other than the self. Bourdieu explains that sections of the aristocracy and the emerging bourgeoisie used their cultural and educational capital – intellectual work and education – to play a pivotal role in the French Revolution. This new class of state nobility, the *noblesse de robe*, differentiated itself from the repressive rule of the aristocracy and monarchies by investing itself in notions of the public and civil service.[10] It made political claims and acted in the name of universal welfare, not self-interested goals, on the grounds that, based on its access to education, it possessed the knowledge and expertise to appropriately speak for all. Thus, a new conversion rule was established: intellectual work and learnedness (cultural capital) as well as education became markers of status (symbolic capital), which then could be turned into the right to govern (political capital).[11]

Invested disinterestedness of the state nobility was, and continues to be, based on the claim to act on behalf of another and to be compelled by something that is greater than the self – "in the form of spontaneity or passion, in the mode of 'it is stronger than me.'"[12] This logic spread into other micro-worlds, such as literary, artistic, and scientific fields. Bourdieu notes that scientists-to-be likely become invested in a disinterested profession in the first place owing to their social position and family origins. He finds that scientists who attended more theory-based schools of higher learning, as opposed to technical scientific colleges, tend to come from families with one or more members who are already part of the scientific field.[13] Hence, invested disinterestedness of the scientist – to pursue knowledge for the sake of knowledge, to be invested in progress and the common good – is not an inherent quality of scientists. Rather, it emerged in a particular historical context in which redistribution of wealth allowed a new social group, the bourgeoisie, to access economic capital that it had not possessed before and to define a collection of virtues that set this new group apart from the aristocracy and the monarchy, with its attendant repression, and from the working class, which the bourgeoisie sought to rule. For the bourgeoisie, having an unfaltering concern for the universal, and beyond the self, was made possible because that group had acquired economic and cultural capital. Being in a dominant position in both the economic and cultural fields provided the bourgeoisie with the luxury to move away from a focus on immediate life necessities and instead to contemplate the universal, common welfare, aesthetics, and the pursuit of knowledge.

To equate invested disinterestedness as a marker of class, however, oversimplifies the concept as a motivation and social norm. For Bourdieu, the concept is specific to the rise of the European bourgeoisie and the particular ethos of this social class. His perspective helps demystify the idea of acting on behalf of another and situate it within social struggles. At the same time, there is a sincerity in invested disinterestedness, through motivation that is tied to feelings of honour. The pursuit of the common good, knowledge, and the health and well-being of others is both genuine and strategic. This tension lies at the heart of the concept of invested disinterestedness, and does not call for a resolution. Invested disinterestedness has within it ties to class struggles that go beyond, but include, the economic and political. At the same time, it includes a genuine motivation to act on behalf of something or someone other than the self, in pursuit of something universal that goes beyond the self. It is a contradiction that is inherent to this game, which denies that it is a game.

Maintaining the Denial

It takes considerable effort to uphold invested disinterestedness and to continuously deny that the game is a game. As much as they rely on economic capital to exist, and to reward invested disinterestedness, anti-economic fields such as scientific, artistic, and religious worlds must always keep economic and other external forces at bay. These fields must be sufficiently autonomous from other fields, particularly the economic field, because, while they rely on economic capital, they also deny this dependence. This balancing act is always to some degree precarious, under threat of falling apart. Bourdieu argues that the scientific field needs to balance two variations of scientific capital – intellectual and bureaucratic – in order to maintain its autonomy.

> Because the autonomy is never total and because the strategies of the agents engaged in the field are inseparably scientific and social, the field is the site of two kinds of scientific capital: a capital of strictly scientific authority, and a capital of power over the scientific world which can be accumulated through channels that are not purely scientific (in particular, through the institutions it contains) and which is the bureaucratic principle of temporal power over the scientific field such as those of minister and ministries, deans and vice-chancellors or scientific administrators.[14]

The "purely scientific" intellectual capital follows the logic of symbolic capital, so that it functions as honour associated with individual scientists based on their recognition from peers for contributing to the pursuit of science for its own sake. In contrast, the "bureaucratic principle" pertains to administrative and funding issues, such as government subsidies to universities, industry funding for research, the political organization of universities, and so on, which are also necessary to do scientific work. Bourdieu asserts that a scientific field in which the purely scientific dominates over the bureaucratic tends to be more autonomous than in a scientific field where the dominance is skewed in the opposite direction. However, autonomy is never complete, and the effects of the bureaucratic principle always loom over the purely intellectual work of science.

Bourdieu finds similar juxtapositions in the journalistic field. There, he argues that there are two spaces – autonomous and heteronomous.[15] Autonomous spaces are where "pure" journalism is done, or where the pursuit of news for democratic visions of reportage is the dominant ethos. Heteronomous spaces of journalism are affected by, and dependent on, economic forces, in the form of audience ratings, advertising revenues, and competition between news agencies for coverage. Journalism is also in a symbiotic relationship with politics and the social sciences. All three fields are involved in, and have stakes in, shaping discourses about political issues and how and by whom these problems should be addressed. Politicians and social scientists rely on media exposure to influence representations of political reality. Politicians and journalists rely on social scientists to provide scientific legitimacy to their position with research data. Finally, journalists and social scientists rely on politicians to implement policy and governmental changes that reflect their own political views. This heteronomous space allows journalists to support their professional visions of democratic debate and political participation, by having non-journalists influence the reporting and shaping of news.

However, the greater and deeper that journalism's symbiotic relationship is with politics and the social sciences, the further that journalism's autonomy diminishes. A result can be that one of these other fields threatens the core tenets of modern journalism, which is to prioritize "pure" journalism, for the sake of democratic values, untainted by economic or political forces. We see this threat today in some major news outlets, where diminished public funding or the purchase of networks by powerful media moguls leads to a greater emphasis on audience ratings, advertising revenues, and sensationalization of news, over and above journalistic integrity. Political leaders can also influence publicly funded networks, through gag orders, censorship, and reportage that favours the ruling party's values.

Similarly, science and medicine have autonomous and heteronomous spaces, where, respectively, either the "purely intellectual" or the "bureaucratic principle" dominates. Yet the solution is not a simple matter of ensuring that the purely intellectual work of science can be done without the interference of bureaucratic forces. The pursuit of science is often expensive, requiring costly technology and labour by researchers, lab technicians, project managers, and human resources coordinators. The disinterested work of intellectual science for its own sake directly relies on a healthy stream of funding and on university bureaucracy, neither of which are entirely disinterested. In order to do their clinical work, doctors in clinics also rely on paid health care managers and health insurance coverage. If they have private practices, then physicians are essentially small-business owners and must contend with overhead costs, hiring and managing employees, and dealing with governmental or other forms of health care insurance. These non-medical, unscientific practices are all necessary bases for the work of "real" science or "real" medicine. This contradiction is at the heart of invested disinterestedness. Although the newly formed bourgeoisie claimed to act in the interest of others and in the name of causes beyond their own interests, these claims were made possible precisely because this class had access to economic and cultural capital – the bourgeoisie had the time and luxury to do disinterested work of public service. Similarly, the scientist is able to claim to be invested in doing science for its own sake and the physician is able to claim to do medicine for the sake of their patients, concerns that transcend the self and immediate necessities, precisely because these necessities have already been secured, through funding and resources to which physicians have access.

Hence, the scientific field can remain autonomous if intellectual work dominates over the bureaucratic principle, at least in appearance, so that the collective denial of the game as a game may continue. Indeed, the very notion of scientists "managing" their conflicts of interest, in the form of affiliations with pharmaceutical companies, for example, is based on the idea that such connections are a necessary evil that needs to be tolerated. Scientists, with their pure intentions and moral integrity, will ensure that market forces will not influence the actual work of science and will protect "pure" scientific intellectualism.

Double Habitus

Scientists and physicians need particular dispositions, sensibilities, and reasoning in order to do science and medicine for their own sake and for the common good, all the while relying on economic products and political forces to enable them to do this work. They need a habitus that corresponds to the precarious and contradictory logic of an anti-economic universe. Broadly, the "habitus" is a set of dispositions of the body and an embodied sense of what is tasteful, possible, and sensible, as well as what is distasteful, impossible, and insensible. From food preferences and taste in art, to moral judgments and ability to wield technical equipment, we develop these dispositions in our bodies and in our minds through our social upbringing and learning in various social worlds, such as our families, communities, schools, the media, religious institutions, the law, and so on. We develop these dispositions in order to play the game to the best of our ability, within the confines and constraints afforded us by the field. Hence, we form our embodied dispositions in direct relation to our position in the field. The kinds and amounts of capital we possess and to which we have access all shape our dispositions. For example, Bourdieu found in his study of French society in the 1970s that the working class prefer hearty foods in hefty portions, an eating practice that likely emerged out of the need to do long hours of manual labour but now has become part of the group habitus. In this way, qualities that feel personal and individual, such as food preferences and taste in art, music, or clothing, are based on our social location and upbringing. In this sense, the habitus is an attribute of an entire social group of individuals who are similarly positioned in a field.

Yet, the habitus is not a predetermined destiny. It functions more as a guide for people of certain social groups on how to play the game to the best of their ability, within the constraints and possibilities that are determined by the field. Rather than being a set of rigid rules of "cannots," the habitus is a wide range of possible thoughts and actions, which are more or less sensible. Hence, people more often think or say "this is more sensible than that," or "that is just silly," than they would think or say "one can/cannot do that." The range of possibilities varies by field and, because most of us partake in multiple games and multiple social worlds, this means that we embody multiple dispositions, sensibilities, types of common sense, and practical knowledge, depending on which games we are playing.

Scientists and physicians are in a unique position, because they play two contradictory games at once – the game of science for its own sake and the game of economics and politics, which makes the game of science possible in the first place, though they can't really talk about that. Bourdieu describes this type of situation as a double habitus. The example he uses as an illustration is priests in the Roman Catholic Church, who claim to do the work of their faith for its own sake, for the benefit of the congregation, and in the name of God, yet who also oversee the operations of their church, which includes calculating the labour of volunteers and employees of the church in terms of monetary value. When it comes to their own contributions to the church, however, the same priests reject the description of their work in terms of labour in the economic sense.[16] The fact that the church is a big business is denied throughout. It is precisely through this collective denial that the economy of the church is able to function primarily as an institution of devotion and faith. Catholic priests are managers of the church, which is a business-denied-as-such, and also do disinterested work of faith and self-sacrifice. In this sense, they must occupy two contradictory habitus: one that corresponds to the economic field and the other that is situated within a highly autonomous area of the religious field. To hold this contradiction in balance, without one habitus subsuming the other, people who simultaneously play contradictory games are guided by a double habitus, which gives them a genuine investment in both games. Hence, priests have a genuine sense of investment in the church as a business, and seek to properly manage the books, but they also genuinely deny that their services are part of this church-as-a-business. Instead, they are genuinely invested in the belief that they – and the church as a whole – are acting primarily in the name of faith and devotion.

Similarly, scientists and physicians possess a double habitus. They have a genuine investment in research funding, health care insurance, competing with other scientists/physicians, managing projects and clinics, dealing with policy makers and university/hospital administrators, and other economic and political aspects of doing science and medicine. At the same time, they genuinely value doing science for its own sake and for the sake of the common good. In the world of scientists and physicians, knowing how to play the game of economics and politics does not fundamentally contradict their claim to do science and medicine in the interest of the public and for the pursuit of knowledge for its own sake. Bourdieu argues that the double habitus is not based on a lie or an illusion but rather that reflects

> a gap between the objective truth, repressed rather than ignored, and the lived truth of practices, and that this lived truth, which hides, through agents themselves, the truth brought to light by analysis, is part of the truth of practices in their complete definition. The truth of the religious enterprise is that of having two truths: economic truth and religious truth, which denies the former.[17]

It is important to note that we cannot explain one motivation in terms of the other. Neither the economic interests of the scientist and the physician, nor their disinterested pursuits of the common good, are the "truer" habitus at work. Both are true at once, in the sense that both motivations are genuine. The double habitus of scientists and physicians allows – indeed, compels – them to repress the fact that their economic/political savvy directly contradicts their disinterested scientific motivations.

Crisis of Faith

Around the repression and denial emerges a range of possible thoughts, actions, and claims that scientists and physicians can draw on when they play the game of science and medicine. For example, when physician scientists explain how they "manage" their conflicts of interest, they repress the fact that their financial affiliations with a for-profit industry fundamentally conflict with the disinterested ideals of their scientific practice. The expression "managing conflicts of interest" is possible in the first place only because scientists and physician possess a double habitus, and the expression in turn serves to reinforce their capacity to repress the truth of their contradictory motivations.

Bourdieu argues that, in disinterested fields, there are terms and expressions whose function is to translate the effects of the economic/political field into language that is suitable for the disinterested field in question. For example, in the religious world of priests, he identifies certain linguistic pairings, such as "apostolate/marketing, faithful/clientele, sacred service/paid labour," that are expression of "two worlds, superimposed on each other as if in a musical chord."[18] The second word in each pair expresses the particular religious practice in economic terms, while the first is its euphemistic equivalent. For those who are not socialized into the religious field and who do not possess the dispositions of a double habitus, these linguistic pairs sound fundamentally deceitful, paradoxical, and hypocritical. Euphemisms allow a double habitus to persist at the discursive level. For example, Bourdieu suggests that the church represses its exploitation of unpaid labour by transforming such work into volunteerism – disinterested work that is its own reward, rather than work that should be compensated, as in the economic field.[19] The euphemism of volunteerism is able to persist because the double habitus of those invested in the field of religion (priests, nuns, elders, people of the congregation, devotees, and so on) and the rules of the religious field allow the linguistic slippage from exploitation to volunteerism as a genuine and natural part of practising religion.

I add to Bourdieu's discussion of repressed truths that those with a double habitus do not necessarily deny the existence of a contradiction altogether – they recognize that what they genuinely believe to be disinterested has economic and political implications. Instead, they repress the non-disinterested truth. The double habitus creates a space between the economic/political truth and the disinterested truth where a person can sit, more or less comfortably, without having a crisis of faith. When scientists claim to manage their conflicts of interest, what they repress is not the fact that scientific work has economic and political implications: this issue is well known, and scientists and physicians often discuss the tension between economic and disinterested forces in their fields. What they do repress is that these two forces are fundamentally incompatible, to the point where it is untenable to hold economic/political and dis-interested motivations at once, without having a crisis of faith. Instead, scientists and physicians, and others who have double habitus, inhabit a mental space where they can suspend their judgment, choose the lesser of two evils, and manage their conflicts of interest. In other words, the field itself creates this space, which allow a distance, discursive and/or bureaucratic, between economic/political truths and disinterested truths, enough so that a person can live in that contradiction. The distance between the two truths harkens back to the lapse of time between the gift and the counter-gift in the village of Kabylia, Algeria. The reason it is taboo for the gift receiver to send a counter-gift too quickly is because the time lapse created a safe distance between the economy of honour and the economy of barter exchange. The distance between the economic/political truth and the disinterested truth – whether it is temporal, physical, symbolic, or bureaucratic – allows an individual to partake in the contradiction.

In science and medicine, as in other anti-economic universes, repressing the contradiction between bureaucratic truth and disinterested truth is not an exception to the rule but rather is at the heart of how invested disinterestedness works. The habitus, and particularly the double habitus, is robust enough to handle the contradiction, especially when the field in question supports the repression of the double truths. The resilience of the habitus is especially marked in Bourdieu's description of the habitus as "a feel for the game":[20]

> Having the feel for the game is having the game under the skin; it is to master in a practical way the future of the game; it is to have a sense of the history of the game. While a bad player is always off tempo, always too early or too late, the good player is the one who *anticipates*, who is ahead of the game. Why can she get ahead of the flow of the game? Because she has the immanent tendencies of the game in her body, in an incorporated state: she embodies the game.[21]

To play the game of science and medicine is to thoroughly embody the game, its rules and stakes, as part of one's being. This includes embracing the rules of scientific method, standards of objectivity, and collegial practice of peer review and critique, and repressing the inherent contradiction between bureaucratic and "purely" disinterested motivations. These technical and moral dispositions are required in anyone who wants to enter the scientific field in the first place. If would-be scientists or physicians had too many doubts or questions about the game and the legitimacy of its rules, then either they would leave the game voluntarily or be rejected from it for being a heretic. If, however, budding scientists or physicians were able to perceive the tension between the bureaucratic and disinterested aspects of science or medicine and tolerate the notion of repressing this contradiction, then they could partake in the game without a crisis of faith. The possibility of dissent and doubt is always there, which is why there are whistle-blowers and revolutions in scientific thought. Yet, as a general rule, such cases are rare and do not result in the dismantling of the entire scientific or medical enterprise. The belief in the possibility of doing science and medicine with objectivity, neutrality, and disinterestedness, despite relying on bureaucratic factors such as funding streams and policies, overrides the possibility of the game being blown out the water entirely.

***

Bourdieu's concept of invested disinterestedness helps identify and qualify the precarious balance in professional medicine between its bureaucratic imperatives (the pursuit of individual livelihood and professional autonomy) and its "purely" disinterested pursuit of knowledge and the common good. The concept also allows us to account for and make sense of how doctors collectively repress this contradiction, as something that can be tolerated because something greater is being achieved. The value of invested disinterestedness as a concept lies in its refusal to resolve this contradiction, compelling the analyst to examine and retain the nuances and idiosyncrasies that often accompany complex situations that require moral decisions. Invested disinterestedness is a useful conceptual and methodological tool for understanding and mapping the moral priorities of medicine, but it should not be thought of as a moral prescription for how doctors ought to act. The very discourse of how doctors ought to act is under scrutiny here, to better understand the broader moral and scientific standards at play that give rise to certain claims about how doctors ought to act. These claims are born out of, and in turn can engender, conflicting ideas about the role and authority of medicine and what it means to be a medical profession and the scope of what it means to "do medicine."

A Brotherhood of Scientific Gentlemen

2

Today's doctors are part of a closely knit professional group. The medical profession demands fierce loyalty from its members, even from potential doctors before they enter medical school. To be a doctor means to adhere to professional codes of ethics, conduct, and patient safety and to subject oneself to the licensing rules of the professional college. In addition to these formal obligations, doctors are socialized to see themselves as part of an elite group, through a competitive admission process for medical schools and then rigorous training in the medical curriculum that tests their intellectual and physical limitations. Regardless of how individual doctors feel about their professional college or association, there is a strong sense among doctors that they are part of a special group with whom they share a unique cultural and professional identity. They are special and elite because of their rigorous training and because the nature of their work puts them in high-stakes positions where their decisions can mean life or death for their patients. Hence, to be a doctor in today's world means to be part of an elite community of like-minded colleagues – one's interest as a doctor is more or less synonymous with the interest of the entire professional group – whose expertise is inseparable from matters of public interest and the common good.

Doctors did not always have, nor did the profession always demand, these internalized feelings of allegiance, camaraderie, and shared identity with other doctors. In the nineteenth century, a period commonly seen by historians as the start of the Canadian medical profession, the profession looked very different from what it is today. In addition to being almost exclusively men, nineteenth-century doctors were largely entrepreneurs, working independently and part of a profession in name only. "Medical men," as they called themselves, openly competed with one another for patients, alongside a plethora of other practitioners who were just as popular as, if not more popular than, licensed doctors. These medical men were internally divided over what constituted appropriate medical education and criteria for entry into the profession, issues that were refracted through broader ethnic and class-based tensions of the period. There was no uniform professional interest to speak of, the public and the state did not trust physicians as an autonomous group of experts, and doctors outright expressed their disdain for the public as an unruly, irrational mob that acted against its own interests by regularly turning to unlicensed and non-medical practitioners. Yet, in a matter of mere decades, medical men went from seeing themselves as more or less independent and disconnected entrepreneurs, with incompatible socio-political differences and conflicting views of what a medical profession should be, to seeing themselves as a united and cohesive brotherhood of scientific gentlemen whose mission was to protect the interest and well-being of the public.

In this chapter, I trace the discursive shifts that shaped the moral and scientific norms of what we know as the medical profession. This early discourse created the foundations on which later claims and statements about the moral and scientific imperatives of medicine were based.

Historical Context

The nineteenth century was a period of change and upheaval for Canadian doctors and their profession. When the British became the dominant colonial regime after defeating the French in 1759, the majority of French medical men returned to France, and those remaining were pushed out to rural areas. British military surgeons and physicians were given automatic licence to practice in the British colony,[1] and, with little competition in a small colonial population, they took over in the urban centres.[2] The first comprehensive medical law after Conquest, the Licensing Act (or the Medical Act) of 1788, drew on a previous bill passed in New France to prohibit anyone who had not successfully passed an examination by a board from practising medicine, surgery, or midwifery.[3] The Medical Act was enforced loosely, if at all. However, during the years immediately following Conquest, this legal laxity did not threaten the dominance of British physicians and surgeons in the medical market.

By the second decade of the nineteenth century, the dominance of British medical men came under threat due to two emerging forces: the rising popularity of non-medical practitioners who began to organize and lobby the government for legislative protection, and the establishment of new medical schools in North America that produced home-grown medical graduates. Most non-medical practitioners were self-taught in various types of healing, which included medicine but also homeopathy, chiropractic, and a new type of botanical medicine called Thompsonian-ism (also called eclecticism). Thompsonians were followers of the work of Samuel Thompson, an American farmer, who had produced a widely popular volume, *New Guide to Health*, in 1822.[4] Thompsonians and homeopaths gained much popularity in the early part of the nineteenth century, particularly among patients who could not afford the services of medical men and also among those who were skeptical of medicine.[5] This was, of course, before twentieth-century scientific medicine, which would dazzle the public with miraculous cures such as penicillin and insulin.[6] The public of the nineteenth century did not have much more faith in the healing abilities of doctors than it did in those of other practitioners. Medical men were frustrated by their competitors but could do little to curb the trend. They were not yet organized into powerful colleges under which they could band together to lobby for greater legislative control of the field. Small groups of medical men in Upper Canada (now Ontario) and Lower Canada (which includes the present-day province of Quebec), and then the United Province of Canada (1841 to 1867), tried to pressure legislatures to give them control over enforcing the medical law and to regulate membership of the profession, but the governments refused to grant medical men legal monopoly over the medical market. Indeed, between 1845 and 1865, medical men proposed a number of bills to the Upper Canada and Lower Canada legislatures with the goal to strengthen medical boards,[7] but, to the great dismay of medical men, the legislature in Upper Canada recognized homeopathy in 1859 and Thompsonians in 1861 as part of the Medical Act.[8]

Added to the challenge of persuading governments, medical men themselves were not united in their vision of what the medical profession should be, and they disagreed with one another on the terms of self-governance. These debates were also happening in Continental Europe, Britain, and the United States, where medical education and certification, the structural organization of professional bodies, the relationship between organized medicine and the state, and the question of what constituted medical knowledge and practice were being configured and reconfigured. The effects of these changes were also felt in Canada, but here they were refracted through social, political, geographic, and economic factors that were specific to nineteenth-century Canada as a British, and formerly French, colony. Most notably, the prevailing understanding that medical men in Canada were British and had been trained in Britain or Continental Europe came under challenge. Until the early nineteenth century, formal Western medical training was available only in Britain and Europe:[9] only those wealthy enough to afford a university education abroad could become doctors. American medical schools were first established in the second and third decades of the century, but, unlike medical schools in Britain and Europe, they were tied to universities and colleges in name only; maintained very loose requirements for courses, theses, and examinations; and generally modified the certification structure relative to student demand, on which the schools relied heavily to pay the faculty.[10] Conservative British medical men in Canada, who sought to emulate the British system of centralized self-regulation and medicine as elite practice,[11] saw the explosion of American medical schools as a threat to this ideal. Meanwhile, the American schools became a popular destination for Canadian students, particularly French Canadians who were predominantly from working-class and rural families and who could not afford to study in Europe.[12] Medical schools were slower to develop in Canada, due to resistance from the imperial government, intent of maintaining its hierarchical relationship to British North America. The Montreal Medical Society (which became the École de Médecine at McGill University) was established in 1824[13] but was not able to grant medical degrees recognized by law until 1834.[14] King's College in York (now Toronto) established its medical faculty in 1839 after years of struggle with the conservative lieutenant-governor from Britain.[15] Outside the coterie of elite British doctors, strong anti-empire sentiments were evident among medical men, particularly among French Canadians, both elite and working class, and working-class British and Americans, as well as medical men of British ancestry born in Canada: none wanted to continue to rely on the empire to train and certify physicians in Canada.

This resistance coincided with non-medical practitioners challenging doctors' monopoly over the medical market. British elite physicians, their years of comfortable dominance threatened, tried to enforce the status quo, resulting in infighting and gatekeeping. Conflicting interests about who belonged in medicine resulted in fundamental debates about what constituted a legitimate medical practitioner and about the role of professional medicine in broader society. None of today's discourse about doctors as an elite group of experts, united under a common professional banner, was readily available at this time. Indeed, a new moral and scientific discourse about what it meant to be a physician emerged in the thick of these conflicts, tensions, and pressures. This discourse revolved around the figure of the gentleman physician, who had unique breeding (i.e., elite class origins) and had cultivated intellect and character (i.e., through medical education at a university). This physician belonged to a brotherhood of gentleman physicians, professionally and emotionally bound to one another in their common pursuit of science and the health of the public. By positioning themselves as guardians of the public's health and the common good, doctors graduated from being a self-interested mass of opportunists to organized professionals with disinterested expertise on which the public could rely. The disinterested habitus of doctors and the definition of the modern medical professional were thus forged in the nineteenth century. The gentleman physician, surrounded by his brotherhood of like-minded colleagues, was at the centre of the medical habitus and embodied the ideals of science and virtue. This figure helped shape and justify both reforms of and restrictions to medical degrees, board examinations, and professional organizations.

The Rational Man

The site of struggle was the question of what counted as legitimate education befitting a gentleman healer. British elite physicians tried to maintain the dominance of a British or European university-based medical education as the only legitimate form of qualification. Meanwhile, non-medical practitioners and graduates of Canadian and American medical schools fought to expand the definition of legitimate medical education to include self-learning and medical degrees that were not from these traditional schools. In response, British elite physicians adopted a joint criteria for what it meant to be scientific and gentlemanly, which in turn provided a new discourse to discredit non-medical practitioners as "quacks" and to monitor undesirable groups and restrict their entry into medicine. The discourse of the gentleman physician brought together specific notions of scientificness and morality: to be scientific was to be rational, to be rational was to be an educated gentleman of particular class standing, and to be a gentleman was to be honourable and trustworthy. This equation worked in both directions, so that being a gentleman from respectable class origins and with appropriate university education meant that a physician was automatically rational and honourable. This equation took some discursive work to develop.

The question of education, or the methods by and conditions under which practitioners acquired their knowledge, was central to the discourse of the physician gentleman. The self-learning model of many non-medical practitioners was a thorn in the side of medical men, who devoted years of study at a university abroad in order to acquire a medical degree. In contrast, the popular text *New Guide to Health* came with a document that certified the reader as a Thompsonian, which meant that anyone could become a practitioner by virtue of purchasing the book. Medical men were extremely hostile to homeopaths and Thompsonians, whose growing popularity threatened their livelihood. One physician lamented in the *British American Journal of Medical and Physical Science* that "under [his] very nose lives neighbour B., who bleeds and extracts teeth at exactly half the professional charge,"[16] calling on the profession to do something about this atrocity.

Although medical men called non-medical practitioners quacks and imposters who preyed on the public, their own knowledge and practices of healing at the time were hardly better than, or even very different, from those of Thompsonians, homeopaths, chiropractors, and other non-medical practitioners. Medicine in the late nineteenth century was not a coherent set of practices that could be clearly set against those of practitioners whom medical men accused of quackery. Medicine at this time consisted of a mishmash of practices based on diverse theories of disease. In Europe, new clinical disciplines, such as anatomy and physiology, were emerging. Meanwhile, in North America an aggressive form of practice came in fashion, which historians have called "heroic medicine." Based on an older conceptualization of health, heroic medicine organized the body in terms of "humours." Illness was caused by an imbalance of bodily humours, and the goal of therapy was to restore bodily equilibrium. Remedies were often aggressive, such as bloodletting using leeches and vomiting induced with purgatives, practices that could lead to death.[17] In heroic medicine, symptoms were the direct and self-evident manifestation of illness.[18] In contrast, the emerging clinical disciplines of anatomy and physiology began to organize the relationship between the body, the cause of disease, and disease symptoms differently. From this perspective, illness was no longer due to an imbalance, but rather could be traced back to a specific locus in the depths and/or surfaces of the body. Symptoms did not indicate illness-as-imbalance as a singular category but could signify a multitude of possible diseases.[19] Clearly, heroic medicine was conceptually more similar to Thompsonianism than it was to medicine influenced by developments in anatomy or physiology. Both heroic medicine and Thompsonianism were based on the principle that "all disease was the effect of one general cause and could be removed by one general remedy" – "cold was the cause; heat, the remedy."[20] At the same time as more-modern approaches to medicine struggled to gain a foothold in Canada, many medical men experimented with Thompsonian remedies as part of their practice, despite the risk of scorn from their peers and even reprimand from their professional body,[21] demonstrating the degree to which heroic medicine, which was the dominant form of medicine during this time, and Thompsonianism were theoretically and practically compatible.

By mid-century, homeopaths and Thompsonians began to petition the elected parliament, the Legislative Assembly of Upper Canada, to include homeopathy and Thompsonianism under medical law. These practitioners used the rhetoric of liberal democracy to attempt to persuade the legislators that they should be given the legal right to practise their craft. A Mr. Flint presented a bill to legalize Thompsonians to the House of Assembly on 5 April 1849:

> [Thompsonians] asked for equal rights but nothing more, they desired the privilege of receiving pay for their services, and if those services were valuable [Mr. Flint] could see no reason why they should not be paid ... In the U.S. the Thompsonian doctors were allowed to practise and the same right should be accorded to them here, to enable them to give their system a fair trial.[22]

Meanwhile, medical men insisted that they themselves be given the authority to enforce the medical law, rather than have the government rely on the hitherto ineffective penal code to punish unlicensed practitioners. The government was not convinced by the arguments of the medical men, and it designated Thompsonianism and homeopathy as part of medicine in an effort to maintain an open medical market that was free of monopoly.[23]

Medical men resisted the perception that their practice was a trade that could be opened up to a market of potential competitors. They insisted that a special kind of preparation and character development were required in order to appropriately administer to the sick:

> The properly educated practitioners, after years of toil and mental exertion, entailing upon him [sic] at the same time a pecuniary outlay, which would form sufficient capital to commence almost any description of business, acquires his Profession, and from his every education scorns to resort to the low chicanery by which the Empiric [a derogatory term meaning charlatan or dishonest practitioner] forces his nostrums upon the ever-gullible public; he treats with contempt the boasted pretensions of the quack.[24]

In the field of medicine, medical men argued, formal education was the only path to moral sensibility and sound medical judgment. The unlicensed practitioner was incapable of these qualities because he was not appropriately trained – that is, educated in a university in Britain or Europe. Hence, a class-based argument linked morality with middle- and upper-class access to medical schooling abroad. Medical men saw Thompsonians and homeopaths, lacking such cultivation of character through appropriate education, as "a set of ignorant and despicable pretenders [who] are to be allowed, by lawgivers, to prey upon society, and sport with human life ... No class of persons can be more devoid of knowledge in science."[25] Physicians protested that "the ignorant pretender" could get away with mistakes and malpractice because a court or a jury could "not presumed to be one whit better informed" about the details of medicine, while "the educated and licensed practitioner, when danger threatens his patient, is required by a sense of moral obligation, by custom and rules of his profession" to seek help and to make a rational decision about whether or not he had made an error.[26] In other words, the educated medical man had the necessary virtues to govern himself because, and only because, he had acquired the appropriate moral dispositions through his professional training, and so he did not need to be subject to an external governance structure such as the penal code.

Meanwhile, the "quack" could not be trusted to self-regulate. The following humorous piece appeared in the *British American Journal*, narrating an interchange between a minister and a homeopath:

> REVEREND GENTLEMAN – Once upon a time I had a cousin, of the name of Thomas Gamble.
> HOMEOPATHIST – And sure enough I am the boy, jist out from Ireland.
> REV. GENT. – And how do you get along, Tom? When I last saw you, you were a Methodist.
> HOMEOPATH. – I now calculate I am a Baptist, and manage to keep my family quite well; I have eighty patients and have cured them all.
> REV. GENT. – Sure, Tom, it is just showing them the physic you are.
> HOMEOPATH. – That is all that is necessary now-a-days, for when they's really sick they don't come to me, but when they fancies themselves sick, I manages to cure them quite readily. They are the best patients; they tries to humbug me, but, I humbugs the cash out of them and that's the point you know.[27]

In this passage, the homeopath not only confesses to deliberately cheating his patients but also admits to having transferred from one religious sect to another, suggesting that he is fickle and lacks integrity. He is also Irish, an ethnic group that was seen as inferior to British and northern Europeans until well into the twentieth century.[28] Finally, he speaks in a manner that betrays his class origin as being below that of the reverend, whom we are assured is a gentleman, although they are cousins. This passage reads as a cautionary tale for medical men that inviting homeopathy and Thompsonianism into the purview of medicine would be the equivalent of having an embarrassing cousin.

Yet medical men could not claim to be superior to the "fraternity of empirics" and the "horde of quacks"[29] simply based on their class origins. Without a clear indication that medical treatments, approaches, and results – their science – were better than those of the so-called imposters, medical men had very little basis for their claims. Indeed, as Thompsonians and homeopaths argued, "Had not many valuable lives been also sacrificed by the regular physician? The only difference was that one [Thompsonians and homeopaths] sacrificed life contrary to law, the other [licensed medical men] according to law."[30] In response to this challenge, medical men invoked a particular kind of scientificness, one that was based on little more than a very general concept of rationality. Medical men based their claims to be scientific on Enlightenment ideals of progress and the genius of the individual. They claimed a historical tradition of medicine that dated back to the ancient Greeks, the originators of all modern Western thought, and the intellectual prowess of physicians as champions of this tradition. As one advocate for doctors observed, "since the time of the deservedly-great *Hippocrates*, centuries before the coming of the Saviour, we trace [the profession's] march, step by step, to its present state of perfection; and very many of the great names in modern history are found enrolled among the faculty – men renowned for their genius and research."[31] Yet Thompsonians, too, drew on Enlightenment discourse – specifically, the democratic value of rationalism – in order to argue that common sense was superior to elite learning.[32] Neither side spoke about medical judgment based in empirical evidence or observation, criteria that characterized scientific medicine of the twentieth century. Instead, the central question was more about the manner in which one acquired the knowledge of medicine and less about the content of the science.

Indeed, science meant something different during this period – in this case, rationality – and standards of scientificness were based on different criteria. In their account of visual objectivity in Western science, Lorraine Daston and Peter Galison demonstrate that, in the nineteenth century, one could claim objectivity by adhering to established and agreed-upon procedures for observation.[33] Scientists could temper any subjective interference by going through rigorous training and cultivating moral and rational competencies that would make them more selfless.[34] For nineteenth-century medical men in Canada, adhering to established procedures meant acquiring university medical education, which they claimed endowed them with the virtues and rational aptitudes that legally and morally qualified them as practitioners of medicine. As one contemporary observer asked, "Who are these 'educated, skillful, and successful physicians?' Are they men who, having acquired their profession honorably, have complied with the requirements of the law in this country, requirements which they well knew, and then quietly settled themselves down in practice; or are they otherwise?"[35]

Medical men claimed that, because they had elite learning, they possessed the moral integrity and scientific competence that are grounded in rationality. They argued, further, that Thompsonians relied on their own interpretations through common sense and, therefore, were incompetent as healers.[36] Medical men often used the words "quack" and "empiric" interchangeably, implying that relying solely on experimentation and observation was both unscientific and immoral compared to basing judgments on formal learning.[37] In this way, medical men sought to reposition Thompsonians' advocacy for common sense as acts of deliberate deception and struggled to establish that elite learning was the only legitimate criterion for scientificness.

Gentlemen Only

The British medical men in British North America extended the argument that elite learning led to scientific rationalism to discredit other forms of medical education. They saw their dominance threatened by medical schools south of the border and by anti-empire sentiments within the colony. These conflicts played out through the medical boards (one in Upper Canada and two in Lower Canada), which examined candidates for a medical licence who had not been educated in a recognized British medical school. Board examiners became gatekeepers of the profession during this time, articulating and implementing certain criteria for the proper scientific and class-based character of a medical man as a way to restrict certain undesirable groups from entering the profession. In doing so, boards articulated the essential qualities of this learned profession – gentlemanliness and scientificness – in terms of the social, political, and ethnic conflicts among medical men in Canada.

Medical boards exercised a considerable amount of power. During the 1820s and 1830s, the board in Upper Canada granted an average of about twenty-five licences per year, while failing candidates on seventy-three occasions between 1830 and 1837 (six of these candidates had applied more than once).[38] Candidates were rejected for three main reasons: disloyalty to the British Crown and lack of integrity (as a single category of defect), deficiency in Latin, and incompetency in anatomy. Demonstration of loyalty was mostly ceremonial, except when it came to American-born candidates, who were required to prove their loyalty and their family's loyalty to Britain during the War of Independence.[39] In general, the board was suspicious of candidates whose families originated in the United States. An early historian of the medical profession in Canada observed:

> After a time, in Upper Canada, there came, now and then, persons from the United States professing to possess medical skill. They came generally, not for attachment to the British flag, but to turn a penny. Sometimes they had a degree of medical education which had been acquired in the United States medical schools; sometimes they knew a little about the use of drugs; but too frequently they only knew how to deceive the people by arrant quackery.[40]

As this quote implies, the medical boards and their supporters conflated loyalty to Britain with qualities of integrity and good moral standing, thereby suggesting that a learned gentleman necessarily had to be pro-Britain.

The same learned gentleman also had to be a cultivated man who had undergone university education, and not someone who was self-taught like a Thompsonian or had attended one of the new privately run schools in the United States. The British considered the latter as opportunistic ventures that profited from tuition rather than emphasizing quality of education.[41] This judgmental stance at times took on a moralized tinge, with references to "the evil and danger of the young men of Upper Canada going to the United States for a medical education."[42] British elite medical men felt threatened by the American medical schools, which allowed greater access to medical training for the middle class, both English and French Canadian, and challenged the elite nature of medicine as the profession of a privileged few. These schools also threatened the goals of British elite medical men in Canada to continue to emulate the hierarchical model of the medical profession in Britain.

Requiring candidates to be proficient in Latin was one way to stave off the threat from self-taught or American-educated applicants. Although medical boards claimed that doctors required Latin in order to write prescriptions and read medical texts,[43] training in the obscure language required a classical university education. This criterion meant that gradu-ates of American medical schools, including many French Canadian candidates, could not pass the medical board examination.[44] The Latin requirement was also a strategy that conservatives in Britain were using in response to a strong faction within the profession that was advocating for reform. Like their counterparts in Canada, the conservatives within the British medical profession maintained that medicine had to be an art of the gentleman and, as such, should uphold classical teachings in universities.[45] Because only those educated at elite public schools and universities would have been taught Latin, the language requirement provided medicine with a sense of exclusivity and eliteness.

By the 1820s, candidates for medical licences in British North Amer-ica were often rejected for incompetency in anatomy,[46] a relatively new subject that was linked to the rise of clinical medicine and hospitals in Europe, particularly in France. Competency in anatomy would have been difficult for graduates of American institutions, who were at a disadvantage owing to a general lack of hospitals and clinical teaching in the country as a whole.[47] The value of anatomy was much debated in Britain at the time. Reformists pushed to include the subject in the medical canon, while conservatives, who sought to maintain a hierarchical separation between surgery and medicine, resisted the move by insisting that the use of hands as required to conduct surgeries on the body was manual labour (the work of the underclass) and not fitting for a learned gentleman.[48] Interestingly, the medical boards in British North America emphasized both Latin, a component of classical education that British conservatives advocated, and anatomy, the new radical subject of the reformists.

Although British elite medical men in the colony tried to emulate the profession as it was practised in their home country, Canada's proximity to the United States meant that the struggle over what was legitimate medical training played out in a different way. In Britain, as anatomy and physiology gained scientific authority, conservatives began to embrace the subjects as legitimate parts of medical education, but only as a supplement to a classical university education.[49] In other words, conservative British medical men used the scientific value of the new medicine to strategically position themselves as simultaneously scientific and gentlemanly. In Canada, Latin and anatomy became ways to maintain British-centrism and to prevent the influence of the American model of decentralized medical education available through for-profit medical schools. These subject requirements also became ways to restrict the entry of French Canadians into medicine, thus further ensuring continued British dominance.

It is curious that medical boards would insist on knowledge of anatomy while medical men in the country were practising heroic medicine, resulting in a situation where two vastly different approaches to medicine, based in entirely different theories of disease, coexisted, and without any apparent problems. Yet this commitment to anatomy was not without limitations: board examinations were verbally administered,[50] an approach that ran contrary to the idea of anatomy as a practical discipline as much as a theoretical one. Clearly, science was deployed strategically and unevenly in order to lend credibility to medical boards, and ultimately to all the medical men inducted via the board as a scientific group of learned gentlemen, while restricting membership of undesirable groups, such as Americans, French Canadians, and radicalized Anglo-Canadians, by claiming that they were both ungentlemanly and unscientific.

Both non-medical practitioners, such as homeopaths and Thompsonians, and the graduates of medical schools in North America threatened the dominance of elite British medical men. The British medical men addressed these threats by restricting what it meant to legitimately practise medicine and what it meant to be a legitimate physician in Canada. This struggle unfolded as a class conflict between the British elite and those who challenged their dominance, but what was also at stake was the definition of scientificness in medicine. Those who challenged the British elite adopted the new democratic discourse of science to argue for an expanded definition of legitimate medical education, one that would include self-learning and non-European medical degrees. In response, the British elite staunchly held onto the importance of medical degrees from British and European medical schools, maintaining that university learning was the only way to ensure that the tradition of rationalism continued in medicine. The two sides strategically deployed different definitions of scientificness in order to lend credibility to their quest to either alter or maintain the existing structural hierarchy in organized medicine. In Canada, the British elite more or less maintained its dominance, setting the groundwork for the modern university-educated medical professional.

Honour among Brothers

Ongoing struggles about who could and could not enter into the profession meant that medical men were often embroiled in arguments and conflicts. Disputes that began with banter could escalate into heated exchanges of ugly insults, some of which were published in medical journals as angry letters. Such internal strife became problematic and embarrassing for medical men, who wanted to convince a reluctant government that they should regulate their own profession and take charge of the medical laws. These public quarrels painted medical men as divided, petty, and unfit to govern themselves – in short, the very opposite of honourable gentlemen. Medical men needed a way to be able to engage in debates – including those about what it meant to be a gentleman physician and who was allowed into the profession – without preventing group cohesion and yet while allowing dissenting individuals to save face. Etiquette became an important governing principle among medical men. It helped regulate not only the large structural conflicts between conservative and reformist positions within the profession, but also contain the everyday spats between medical men when they competed with one another for patients. At first, the informal rules of conduct and professional etiquette around how to treat one another were messy and inconsistent, but they eventually stabilized into a coherent discourse of brotherly feeling toward other gentleman physicians. This discourse worked only if medical men fully embodied the feeling of being connected to other medical men in a brotherhood that collectively strove for the highest standards of scientificness and gentlemanly honour.[51] Medical morality during the nineteenth century focused on the idea that physicians ought to behave honourably toward fellow physicians, to the point where being a physician would automatically mean being inculcated into a brotherhood. Indeed, the first code of ethics of the Canadian Medical Association in 1868 devoted more pages to detailing the rules of professional etiquette than to explaining physicians' obligations to their patients and the public. Over the course of the century-long conflict over who could legitimately be a physician, there was a marked shift in how medical men approached questions of honour. They went from being focused on defending their own personal honour to protecting the honour of the whole professional group, marking an important shift away from competition and self-motivated interests and toward the disinterested ethos of a professional group.

The nineteenth century saw major shifts in the cultures of Europe and its colonies, including in codes of masculinity among white European men. As monarchies and much of the aristocratic class was dismantled, the new class of the bourgeoisie emerged and along with it new codes of masculinity. Bourgeois men carved out spaces to which they had exclusive access, such as gentlemen's salons and clubs, as part of their classed and gendered identity. However, it was unfashionable to blatantly discriminate based on class and ethnicity during a time when the Enlightenment ideals of democracy dominated the cultural mood in Europe and its colonies. Robert Nye argues that bourgeois men adapted the concept of the duel as a way to monitor membership in the gentlemen's clubs. In particular, bourgeois men wanted to bar the entry of women and certain types of undesirable men (such as working-class and Jewish men).[52] By the nineteenth century, duelling was perceived as archaic, flashy, and spectacle-driven, typical of the aristocracy and antithetical to the values of restraint of the new bourgeoisie. However, the ethical framework of the duel – to respond to an insult with a challenge that would give one the opportunity to defend one's integrity and honour – appealed to bourgeois men. Nye argues that bourgeois men adopted the ethic of the duel without engaging in the actual physical act of fighting, which allowed them to resolve disputes in a manner that distinguished them from the old aristocracy. Adapting a practice that belonged to the former ruling class also allowed bourgeois men to distinguish themselves from the working class. The rules of duelling-without-the-duel provided an ethical framework for white European men, including scientists and physicians, to deal with interpersonal conflict, such as scientific debates at conferences and symposia, which sometimes escalated to personal attacks, in a manner that is still consistent with middle-class values of restraint.

Duels with words between physicians appeared in the editorial pages of medical journals throughout the nineteenth century. Medical men attacked one another's character and integrity, which they conflated with scientific merit and political opinions. In this editorial sparring, medical men outlined the terms and criteria for gentlemanly conduct that were fitting for a physician as a way to challenge and discredit their opponents. A particularly heated dispute appeared in the pages of the *Dominion Medical Journal* in 1868 between "Dr. Yates," a former member of the Upper Canada Medical Council,[53] and "Dr. Fields," another member of the council, over the matter of Thompsonians and homeopaths. When the government of the United Province of Canada passed an amendment to the Medical Act to legalize homeopathy 1859, a few medical men suggested that they embrace these practitioners in order to directly influence them and thereby weed them out, an approach that one physician described as "hugging eclectics [i.e., Thompsonians] to death."[54] Yates wrote to the editor of the *Journal* to describe why he supported this view, stating that there were bound to be "knaves and fools" in any profession, including medicine, and that such inferior "rascals" could be relegated to the lower status of homeopaths and Thompsonians, which are "two bastard branches of medicine."[55] Fields, who was one of five homeopaths elected to the Upper Canada Medical Council after the amendment of the medical law, took great offence at Yates's use of derogatory terms to describe his homeopathic colleagues, and accused Yates of being ungentlemanly. The subsequent exchange between the two men was about how one could claim to be a gentleman. Yates and Field agreed that a gentleman "may attack any system or doctrine which he believes to be false or dangerous, but must avoid personal or individual abuse."[56] Paradoxically, both men used personal attacks in order to accuse the other of not upholding these ideals, and neither referred to the flaws in the medical theories or remedies of their opponent's profession. Nye explains that, in the old rules of the duel, what mattered was not so much who was in the right as who was "willing to back up his words with deeds" – to challenge an opponent to a duel.[57] In the absence of physical aggression, Yates and Field backed their respective positions by calling on various qualities of a gentleman, qualities that they then claimed the other was lacking. By discrediting their opponent, the two men sought to elevate their own position as in the right.

Yates versus Field was a personal conflict between two men, very much in the style of the duel, rather than a disagreement between two groups of practitioners with different approaches to illness and remedy. Another approach to engaging in conflict emerged during the nineteenth century, one that still maintained gentlemanly honour but that specifically appealed to the honour of the entire professional group. This shift was most notable in the conflict between British elite and French Canadian medical men in Quebec at mid-century. In 1846–47, there were several significant organizational and legislative changes in medicine in Quebec. In 1847, the province established a College of Physicians and Surgeons, a governing body that followed the British model, and made numerous attempts to revise the provincial medical act. French Canadian medical men felt excluded by the British, who spearheaded both initiatives, and accused the latter of illegally naming a college without the input and support of all physicians. British elite medical men responded with insults, dismissing the French for irrationally resisting a process that would ultimately benefit them and called their actions a "fitful phantom of a disordered mind."[58] The British also accused the French of being jealous of those in power and of acting selfishly to "assert a Franco-Canadian supremacy over the Anglo-Canadian or British,"[59] combining personal insult with the patronizing expressions of superiority of the British toward the French.

This dispute was as heated as the quarrel between Field and Yates, but in it we can see indications of group interests, rather than a resort to impugning the personal integrity of a single individual. In 1846, a contingent of medical men from the École de Médecine at McGill University had objected to a medical bill that was being drafted by a group of British doctors. The bill required McGill graduates to undergo examinations by the medical board in order to obtain a licence to practice, while the graduates of recognized schools in Britain were to be granted automatic licences. A five-page editorial in the *British American Journal of Medical and Physical Science* contained criticisms of the McGill contingent for obstructing the legislation, arguing that the school faculty acted in a misguided self-interest that ran contrary to the "dearest and best interests of the community at large."[60] The editor, who was evidently sympathetic to the British elite, portrayed the McGill contingent as a hostile minority and represented the interests of the profession in terms that clearly favoured the position of British medical men. While claiming that the matter "must be viewed through no distorting medium of prejudice, or passion, or interest," the editor suggested that, "if we can make it appear that the interests of the profession generally ... are the interests which would be really affected by the concession of the power which the School of Medicine is demanding, it will then follow ... that the School of Medicine is pursuing a course of policy which is hostile to the best interests of that profession from which it claims its support."[61] And in this goal, he claimed, *"a large, a very large, majority of the British practitioners of Canada,* who desire to see their profession placed on some more elevated and stable position than it now occupies, will fully sustain us."[62]

The editor's personal bias is undeniable. He claimed unbiased judgment but was clearly appealing to the interests of his British colleagues. This was a calculated move to discredit the French by portraying their position as self-interested and irrational, while implying that the British medical men were the vanguard of medical disinterestedness and rationality. Aside from the blatant attempt to shape the medical profession in terms of British interests, the editor also opened up the possibility of discrediting the French opposition without having to resort to individualized insults. Individual sparring, as in the dispute between Field and Yates, was often passionate, irrational, and, therefore, unscientific. The editor deferred to the rational judgment of medical gentlemen as a group, which was dominated by the British, to conclude that the French opposition was self-interested, and therefore unprofessional, not disinterested, unscientific, and ungentlemanly. The message was that, to be honourable was to maintain rational poise and speak on behalf of the entire professional group, rather than shout from the margins. By foregrounding gentlemanliness as a sign of professionalism, the British elite doctors could dismiss the opposition from their French counterparts on the grounds that the latter were acting in an ungentlemanly fashion, without having to resort to petty arguments and attacks.

By adopting the ethics of the duel, medical men were able to engage in struggles and disagreements about fundamental issues, including professional governance and legitimate means of becoming a member of the profession, in a manner that was aligned with the emerging discourse of the bourgeois gentleman. However, disputes between gentleman physicians generated internal tensions and put the entire group in a negative light in the eyes of the public and the state. By appealing to the interests of the group instead, medical men not only settled internal disputes over professional matters, but they also gave shape to the idea of the medical profession as an entity with a set of identifiable interests and an honour that its members had to defend. The shift from defending one's personal honour to protecting the honour and interests of the group opened up the possibility of imagining medical men as a cohesive and united profession.

Family Feeling

For medical men to unite as a profession, they needed to feel that they belonged to a profession with other medical men. In Bourdieu's words, they needed to "give a candle" about their colleagues, and not just see them as other physicians or business competition. Medical men needed to see other medical men as fellow members of a profession, with whom they shared goals and interests. They also needed to genuinely feel that an attack on the professional group was an attack on their own self, and that for an individual member to act dishonourably or in his own self-interest was to hurt the honour of the entire group. This group ethos and feeling organized around the concept of brotherhood. As brothers, medical men had to value the group over and above the self, even during moments where they engaged in disputes about professional governance and medical opinions and competed with one another for patients. This meant that they had to feel a genuine and powerful affective bond with their colleagues, and this feeling had to be rooted in an embodied sense of honour, trust, and familial connection. Creating these feelings required considerable work, and writings in medical journals at this time were filled with details about what this brotherly feeling looked like. Specifically, there was considerate effort in these writings to connect honour, status, and scientific merit under a single rubric of a professional ethos – the brotherhood of gentlemen doctors.

Open competition and a private practice model were the greatest obstacles to establishing affective bonds of brotherhood among medical men. In between the dramatic episodes of higher-level disputes about professional governance were more frequent petty squabbles and clashes related to daily work. Some of these instances were patient driven. For example, a physician might be called to a patient's home for an emergency only to find, on arrival, that the patient had also summoned another physician. Some situations were physician-driven, such as where a physician deliberately interfered with another's relationship with his patient by offering contradictory medical advice. There was no formal code of conduct about how to deal with such embarrassing and unpleasant situations. Writings in medical journals at this time reported on such incidents and emphasized that medical men had to honour the bonds of brotherhood with others in the profession. Instead of seeing a neighbouring physician as a potential rival or competitor, a medical man who was a true gentleman dedicated to his craft would be guided by an "honourable feeling"[63] and a respect for "the feelings and opinions of others,"[64] so that he would see a fellow medical man as a "brother practitioner."[65] The first code of ethics of the Canadian Medical Association, published in 1868, reinforced the familial feeling by insisting that medical men had to provide care for another's family free of charge and that they should, in turn, had a right to expect such service from their fellow medical men.[66] The rationale was that, if physicians saw one another as brothers in a professional family, then they would naturally uphold professional etiquette, maintain the familial feeling as a default affective state, and embody the rules of gentlemanly honour as their innate moral compass. Ideally, physicians would be driven by an internalized rule that did not feel like a rule, so that they would not be able to imagine overstepping the bounds of their practice to infringe on that of another physician, and they would feel genuinely uncomfortable when another physician's patient requested a consultation.

However, a genuine feeling of brotherliness toward other physicians conflicted, at times, with the reality that debate is part of the social practice of medicine as science. Even if medical men felt honour bound to one another, they were inevitably going to have diverse opinions on medical judgment, and, as scientists, physicians were likely to engage in disputes in ways that could compromise brotherly feelings. In a two-part series on medical ethics, W. Fraser wrote in the *British American Journal of Medical and Physical Science* about various situations in which medical men might find themselves at odds with one another. Specifically, he referred to a situation where a physician suspected that the life of a patient of another physician was in danger as a result of an error in medical judgment. Quoting Thomas Percival, a conservative British physician and an authority on medical ethics,[67] Fraser stated that the physician had the duty to interfere, so long as the information on which he based his intervention was "well founded" and "his motives are pure and honorable."[68] In another instance, Fraser referred to the words of a colleague who insisted that interference was inappropriate in any situation because good intentions are not enough. The intervening medical man "will almost infallibly be regarded with a suspicion of self-conceit, which ... a rightful minded man would avoid, as calculated to injure his character and impair his usefulness."[69] The first position looked to the physician's intentions in order to assess whether or not a medical judgment was honourable, while the second cautioned that the perception of dishonour could override the individual's intentions. At the end of the editorial, Fraser was undecided as to whether the suspecting physician was justified in interfering.

What is particularly interesting about Fraser's ethical dilemma is the emphasis in the second position on others' perception of a behaviour as (dis)honourable, regardless of one's intentions. Writers in medical journals on the subject of professional decorum focused on how disputes and arguments between medical men, however well meaning and respectful, could discredit the profession in the eyes of those outside of medicine, namely, patients, the public, and legislators. These writers depicted a medical man's lack of professional etiquette as simultaneously unbrotherly and unscientific: "Every injury thus inflicted on the individual ... is felt by the profession at large, of which he is a member ... It cast[s] discredit and disrepute on scientific practice."[70] Even legitimate scientific debates could be misunderstood as dishonourable and could "degrade the profession in the eyes of the public,"[71] an outcome that dishonoured not only the individuals involved but, more importantly, the entire professional group. If medical men were to lose credibility as a profession for being divided, this could compromise their efforts to acquire greater autonomy and to oversee the medical law.

The Canadian Medical Association's first code of medical ethics in 1868 placed much emphasis on the impact that the ways in which medical men acted toward one another could have on public perceptions of the group as a whole. Referring specifically to private practice, the code advocated that medical men strive for consistency and unity across the group, so that they could transform the prevailing public perception that they were rivals in a competitive medical market into a perception that they were a profession of colleagues who supported one another. For example, in the code, wealthy medical men were asked not to undercharge a patient, because "his doing so is an injury to his professional brethren."[72] It also recommended that all medical men refrain from advertising because it was "derogatory to the dignity of the profession."[73] These sections of the code emphasized that medical men needed to be conscious about promoting honourable feeling as an identifiable quality of the group, in order to advance a sense of the respectability and credibility of individual physicians, and of the entire group, among the public at large.

Nevertheless, disagreements and arguments were bound to occur between physicians. Part of their role as scientists was to engage in debate and to critique and challenge ideas with rigour. As clinicians, they had to be able to verify and review their own medical judgment, including that related to diagnosis and appropriate remedies, but they also might be called on to make such assessments about another physician's medical judgment, as in Fraser's ethical dilemma discussed above. And such assessments were likely to generate conflict, however minute or grand in scale. Even when the parties involved had the highest respect for one another, an outsider who was not part of the professional group could construe a legitimate scientific debate as a petty quarrel and a questioning of character. Thus, handling public perceptions of internal conflicts within the profession was as important as cultivating honourable feelings of brotherhood among medical men themselves. The first concerned the appearance of credibility, while the latter related to internal cohesion, and physicians needed both to secure the reputation of the profession as a united group of experts whom the public and the government could trust to be honourable.

The code of ethics repeatedly highlighted the importance of dealing with debates, disputes, and conflicts behind closed doors and away from the public eye. During a consultation, all the attending medical men should "retire to a private place for deliberation" and then discuss the case with the patient "in the presence of all the faculty attending"; nothing should be discussed "which are not the result of previous deliberation and concurrence."[74] By conducting deliberations in private, the consulting medical men should present to the patient an appearance of cooperation and confidence in the medical judgment, while concealing any possible unpleasantness and differences of opinion that might have arisen during the discussion. The code elaborated:

> As peculiar reserve must be maintained by physicians towards the public, in regard to professional matters, and as there exist numerous points in medical ethics and etiquette through which the feelings of medical men may be painfully assailed in their intercourse with each other, and which cannot be understood and appreciated by general society, neither the subject-matter of such differences nor the

adjudication of arbitrators should be made public, as publicity in a case of this nature may be personally injurious to the individuals concerned, and can hardly fail to bring discredit to the faculty.[75]

This passage warned medical men not to air their dirty laundry in public because a person who was not trained in medicine would not possess the embodied sense that there were times when scientific debate about medical judgment could lead to less honourable interactions between medical men. An outsider would not realize that seemingly dishonourable interactions did not mean that the parties involved had dishonourable intentions. Medical men possessed the know-how and common sense that allowed them to see that such tensions were an inevitable part of medical practice. However, the public did not understand this nuance. Thus, for physicians to engage in open debate in front of a patient could reveal this contradiction and risk the group being perceived as incompetent, rather than engaging in a proper scientific process.

For medical men to create a veneer of consistency and confidence, they needed to demarcate private and public domains that were clearly distinguished from one another. In the private space behind closed doors, they could conduct their internal affairs, where individual physicians could present their own arguments with respect to scientific debates and professional governance. Then, in the public space outside these doors, they could present the conclusions and decisions of the entire group to the patient and the public. Family feeling toward other medical men, and indeed the entire profession, reinforced the need for private space in which the profession could air its disagreements, debates, and grievances.

On Behalf of Public Interest

By organizing their moral code around the need to defend the honour of the professional group, rather than to save their own face, medical men created the notion that they were part of a brotherhood of gentlemen who were honour-bound to one another. However, for them to claim a moral high ground in comparison to the "quacks" and to win the trust of the government in their quest to dominate the medical market, they needed to do more than display honour toward one another. Medical men needed to demonstrate that they could also be counted on to defend the interests of those outside their professional group. Here, the public became the ideal external object that gave moral credibility to physicians. Physicians could claim to be disinterested by demonstrating that they were acting primarily on behalf of the interests of the public, not themselves. The cholera epidemics of the early nineteenth century provided an ideal historical context in which medical men could shape the discourse of public health in terms of the moral and ethical obligations of physicians to protect the interests and health of the public.

The concept of "the public" is relatively new, emerging in the nineteenth century in direct relation to the changes in governing and statecraft in Europe during this time. Michel Foucault has written about the emergence of different types of sovereign power in European history and how the significance of the notion of "the people" changes vis-à-vis shifting organization of sovereign power.[76] He argues that a new approach to governing emerged in the nineteenth century, replacing the repressive monarchy/oligarchy with the managerial nation state. While the monarch had previously dealt out repression and capital punishment in the exercise of his or her sovereign power, the new state was interested in maintaining a healthy and productive population. The "population," unlike the unruly mob, had desires, opinions, biological realities, and economic functions that the state had to contend with and at times appease. Under the managerial state, a plethora of expert discourses and practices proliferated, such as psychiatry, the penal system, and clinical medicine, in order to understand the population and maximize its productivity. In *The Birth of the Clinic*, Foucault argues that medicine acquired a positive significance – as opposed to the negativity of its association with disease and death – by linking up with the state as an apparatus of monitoring and managing the life of populations in a form of governance that he calls "biopolitics."[77] Interestingly, the notion of "the public" appears in Canadian medical journals during the nineteenth century. These writings show two different ways of representing the public – as an irrational mass of patients who cannot distinguish between good and bad medicine, and as an entire population with a collective right to proper medical care. As physicians moved toward the latter discourse, they not only entrenched the public as an object of medical knowledge, but they were also able to claim that the profession was acting in the interest of public health.

Medical men initially developed a protectionist discourse to describe their relationship to their patients and to the public at large. Although physicians claimed that they were scientifically and morally superior to alternative practitioners, the fact of the matter was that their patients saw them as no different from Thompsonians and homeopaths, and at times even preferred these other practitioners. To explain the public's distrust of medicine, medical men described their patients as a group with unpredictable tendencies and temperaments that worked against its own interests. Physicians portrayed the public as irrational and ignorant – "the ever-gullible public"[78] – unable to make sound judgments when it came to selecting the most competent healing practitioner. The public so conceived was vulnerable to imposters and false promises. The quack was equally irrational and ignorant, owing to a lack of proper education and training, and was also dishonourable, preying on the ignorance of the public and wilfully deceiving them: as an early medical historian put it, the quack "would adopt habit and cunning that respectable men could not think of."[79] The medical man was rational, educated, and honourable, and thus could, and, indeed, was obligated to, protect the public from quacks. This argumentative logic transformed the public's healthy skepticism toward medicine into a disregard by an ungrateful public of the honourable intentions of medical men: "if the physician, despite the most judicious application of his talents, cannot arrest the behest of Providence, immediately he is blamed, censured, and even accused!"[80] By extension, the quack's popularity could be explained only as luck: "Their modesty prevents them from trumpeting their own praises, but their good fortune makes others do it for them."[81] The protectionist discourse placed medical men on the defensive, as victims of unchecked quackery and distrust by an irrational, ungrateful mob of patients.

During the cholera epidemics of the 1830s, a new discourse emerged that portrayed patients as a population with rights and interests that required defending by an honourable and benevolent expert body – the medical profession. Medical men claimed that "the public at large has an equal interest" in the competency of any practitioner, be he a medical man or a Thompsonian, and "has a right to expect"[82] that he knows what he is doing. This position was markedly different from overtly condescending descriptions of the public. This new public had interests and rights, and those who claimed to act on its behalf were expected to uphold these entitlements. The public health discourse still maintained the notion that the public was vulnerable to quackery and incompetence because it lacked expert knowledge and training to recognize legitimate medical care. Rather than lament and insult this lack, physicians suggested that medicine not only had the expertise to intervene but that medical men had the moral duty to do so in the name of the public good. By claiming to act on behalf of public interest and to uphold the public's right to competent medical practice, medical men could more successfully claim that their disinterested expertise naturally and ethically obligated them to intervene in matters of public health. And, by this discursive logic, it would be unethical and immoral for them to do nothing in the face of such a grave medical catastrophe as a cholera epidemic. The rhetoric of public health also gave medical men the language to discredit non-medical practitioners and claim moral superiority, without having to resort to pettiness or overt paternalism toward patients.

By positioning themselves as guardians of public health, medical men could participate in governance with much greater credibility. During the cholera epidemics, public health developed as a part-state/part-medical institution, allowing physicians to carve out a more definitive moral and expert role for professional medicine in state governance. Although medical responses to the epidemics revealed deep inadequacies in medical science and divisions among medical men,[83] physicians navigated the terrain of scientific uncertainty and government instability in interesting and productive ways. Linsey McGoey argues that scientific uncertainty is not necessarily always detrimental for scientific experts. Uncertainty can be generative – it can breed new theories and practices to remedy the problem. Also, experts who point out the uncertainty are in a better position to suggest solutions because they are the ones who recognized that a problem exists in the first place.[84] During the cholera epidemics, medical men identified the lack of effective sanitation and hygiene as the source of the problem.

They claimed that boards of health were neglecting public health by ignoring their own laws on sanitation.

> We ask the question, should we not be prepared for its [i.e., cholera's] arrival? Should no sanitary precautions be observed? And finally, is it the proper time to adopt them when the disease has manifested itself, and its virulence has been aggravated by the dirt and filth which furnish a nidus for its incubation and its propagation, and which might have been removed at a more opportune period. Yet opposed to common sense and ordinary reason, as would be the negative answers to these questions, the Executive authorities are acting upon these presumptions.[85]

Although the medical profession was not popular among the public during this time, neither were the boards of health, which had very limited power to enforce public health laws and whose conflicts with medical men were perceived by the public as part of their ineffectiveness. In this vacuum of reliable expertise, medical men positioned themselves as expert advisers to lawmakers in the name of public welfare, thereby claiming their entry into the political arena.

The discourse of public health and acting on behalf of public interest did not resolve the thorny issue of payment. When faced with the imminent threat of Thompsonians and homeopaths becoming licensed under the Medical Act in Upper Canada, medical men scrambled to guard their livelihood in ways that contradicted their protectionist stance in relation to the public. Medical men in rural areas, in particular, lamented that unlicensed quacks undercharged patients and threatened their medical practice to the point of infringing on their rights as licensed practitioners.[86] In a debate in the Legislative Assembly about a government bill to license alternative practitioners, one doctor claimed that the medical man's "bill, always unwelcome, is greeted with a frown; it is paid, when at all, years after, and with a very liberal deduction!"[87] Statements such as this made explicit what must remain implicit in disinterested acts, as described by Bourdieu in relation to gift giving: for an act to be recognized as honourable and not self-interested, there must be an implicit and unspoken agreement between the doer and receiver that the act will be acknowledged and reciprocated through gratitude. Physicians' complaints about not being paid appropriately and in a timely manner exposed this implicit agreement, stripping the act of its honour and disinterested value. When two medical men were denied their request for compensation for serving on the Board of Health in Upper Canada while two of their other colleagues had been compensated, the two unpaid physicians published angry editorials in a medical journal, claiming that they "consider honor and pecuniary emolument, alias 'sweets of office,' to be intimately blended."[88] The public may have had the right to expect knowledgeable and honourable experts to protect them from quackery and malpractice as much as from disease, but medical men would honour this right if and only if the public reciprocated with respect and payment: "As a question of equity, the public have no right to services which its members may not individually claim without paying for them."[89] While physicians may acted in the interests of the public, their services were not instances of self-sacrifice per se. Physicians would honour the public's interest if the public in turn honoured medical expertise and moral duty with payment. Thus, the notion of "the public" provided professional medicine with a way to legitimize itself as a disinterested institution and group, but there was a limit in the extent to which physicians were willing to be disinterested and honourable. Public interest was to be held in tension with professional interest, a precarious balance that would tip in the mid-twentieth century, when the medical profession resisted publicly funded health care.

***

The early medical professional ethos of the nineteenth century was built around the trope of the gentleman, whose ethnic and class-based heritage and access to medical education became synonymous with the ideal qualities of a medical man. This figure was the focal point around which a moral and ethical system developed to deal with the internal conflicts within the burgeoning medical profession and the profession's struggle to discredit other practitioners and dominate the medical market. The gentleman physician had a university education and embodied ideals of rationality and professionalism, and the latter entailed a bourgeois restraint from debasing himself or his gentleman brothers by engaging in petty self-interested conflicts. The idea – and feeling – of a brotherhood of physicians, connected to one another as a profession by an unspoken familial bond, was iterated, repeated, and embedded in the professional discourse of medicine. Through this symbolic and cultural work, those in dominant positions in the profession sought to change doctors' perception of themselves, from a band of self-serving entrepreneurs to a member of a closely knit profession whose moral imperative included protecting the integrity of the profession.

The medical profession justified its claims to be superior to other practitioners, or "quacks," by claiming to act in the interest of public health. The public, a concept that took shape in the nineteenth century, provided professional medicine with a rationale and anchor for its claim to medical disinterestedness. Doctors claimed to practise medicine and advise the government on matters of public health for the greater public good. However, their motivations were not pure altruism or charity. Doctors expected to be paid and to be recognized and respected for their expertise. They sought to be granted the autonomy to control the conditions of their work and medical licensing structures. This unspoken economic and political trade-off for doctors' efforts to protect and promote public health went largely unquestioned until the mid-twentieth century, when the government of Saskatchewan proposed the nation's first state-administered health insurance model, as will be discussed in the next chapter.

Building Bridges, Making Amends   3

Nineteenth-century medical men claimed to be defenders of the public interest in matters of health and illness, but, when it came to the issue of payment, they revealed a limit to which they were willing to act in the service of the public. In this sense, medical disinterestedness was not entirely altruistic. Medicine would act on behalf of the public as long as the public respected doctors' professional interests to be acknowledged and respected as primary experts in matters of health and illness, to be able to determine the conditions of their work, without intervention by the state, and to be appropriately paid for their services. This unspoken understanding underpinned doctors' pledge to honour their patients and the interests of the public as part of their professional mandate. Doctors had a distinct professional interest that was separate from the interests of the public, one that did not become an issue in the everyday business of medicine so long as both parties held up their end of the understanding. This understanding unravelled in the mid-twentieth century, when the medical profession rejected the Saskatchewan government's proposal for tax-funded, state-administered universal health insurance to replace the fee-for-service model.

On 1 July 1962, Saskatchewan doctors walked out of their practices in protest of the new provincial Medical Care Act. Leading up to this event, there had been mounting tensions and resentment between the

Saskatchewan government, led by the Co-operative Commonwealth Federation (CCF), and the medical profession, led by an unprecedented coalition of the Saskatchewan Medical Association (an interest body of the profession) and the Saskatchewan College of Physicians and Surgeons (a regulatory body). When the CCF government opened negotiations with doctors with respect to the new act, the medical profession insisted on a modified version of the existing fee-for-service model, in which the state would provide some assistance through taxation plans for those who could not pay for medical services, and an independent commission, with representation from the college, would administer this plan.[1] The government argued otherwise. It pushed for an entirely prepaid insurance plan, which would be controlled by the state, with doctors becoming salaried government employees.[2] Ever since Premier Thomas C. ("Tommy") Douglas announced in 1959 his party's intention to establish a universal prepaid health insurance plan in Saskatchewan, the two sides had negotiated in meeting after meeting but could not reach an agreement. The negotiations ultimately reached a stalemate, and in November 1961 the government passed the new Medical Care Act without the agreement of the medical profession.

After eight additional months of unsuccessful negotiations, doctors in the province closed their offices en masse, backed by the medical profession,[3] which was confident that these actions would force the government to repeal the act. The press in Saskatchewan had skewed the coverage of the negotiations in favour of the profession, so that the medical profession was by and large under the impression that it had the support of the public.[4] Yet, when the doctors walked out of their clinics and offices and the news went nationwide, national media and the press in other provinces denounced the doctors' actions as an illegal strike.[5] The public demonstration in front of the Parliament Building in Regina on 11 July to support the doctors drew five thousand protesters, less than a fifth of the twenty-five to fifty thousand expected.[6] The strike ended with a negotiation between the medical profession and the CCF government and the signing of the Saskatchewan Agreement, which legalized tax-funded universal medical insurance but still allowed doctors to charge a fee for service on a voluntary basis.[7] Despite reaching a favourable compromise with the government, the medical profession continued to face an angry public, which saw the profession's actions as selfish and elitist.

The walkout by Saskatchewan doctors in 1962 not only was the first doctors' strike in Canada, but the circumstances surrounding this event marked the first time that a government in Canada successfully challenged the medical profession's authority, and also the first time that the medical profession in Canada had encountered public criticism in the media about its integrity. Even before 1 July, and before the intense national and international criticism against the Saskatchewan medical profession, there were concerned murmurings among doctors in Canada that the profession was losing the faith of the public. As twentieth-century medicine became more specialized and scientifically rigorous, the profession faced complaints about being impersonal, lacking compassion, and charging too much. Against this backdrop of increasing public unhappiness with and disapproval, professional medicine was faced with conflict between its interest to control the conditions of doctors' work and the political interest of the CCF government to intervene in health care, as well as the media interest to report on the public's disapproval of the medical profession. Enmeshed in the profession's disputes with the government over payment structure were also differing definitions of health, as the two sides vied for the disinterested position of acting on behalf of the public and its health.

In the process of negotiating with the state and the media, doctors began to question whether an aggressive pursuit of medical science, at the expense of maintaining a close relationship with the public, created a rift between professional medicine and the public. It was the first time since its inception that professional medicine had had to directly deal with the possibility that its scientific interests could conflict with its moral obligations toward the public. Public and media responses to the strike confirmed the existing suspicion among Canadian doctors that their moral legitimacy was in jeopardy. The disastrous aftermath of the walkout spurred the medical profession in Canada to examine its priorities and practices in order to try to repair its damaged relationship with the public. The profession began to prioritize more social and humanistic approaches, namely public health and general practice, but in very specific ways that aligned with medicine's existing scientific goals. The profession also embraced public relations and media work. Initially, the profession had considered these deceptive and antithetical to medical disinterestedness, but they were eventually incorporated into professional practice. Hence, the Saskatchewan affair of the 1950s and 1960s resulted in doctors doing medicine differently in order to regain moral legitimacy.

Defining Health

The standoff between the medical profession and the CCF government in Saskatchewan on the issue of health insurance was a battle between giants. At stake was how the health of the population would be defined, qualified, and insured, as well as who would safeguard it and, therefore, have mastery over it – the state or the medical profession. By the mid-twentieth century, the medical profession was the leading expert body on matters of health and illness. The CCF formed the first socialist government in North America when it became the governing party of Saskatchewan in 1944. These two giants clashed in the arena of health over questions of how health care, including doctors' services, would be paid for, questions that the two sides answered from different understandings of health.

The medical profession argued that the health of a person was achieved within the private relationship between a patient and the attending physician. The doctor-patient relationship was an age-old model of medicine that dated back to times before doctors professionalized in the nineteenth century. At the centre of this model was the entrepreneurial physician, whose private practice served the middle and upper classes through a patronage system. As a point of contrast, by the mid-nineteenth century, doctors who worked in public hospitals provided care for the working class, the poor, and immigrants, as was the case during the cholera epidemics.[8] When the medical profession in Saskatchewan argued against the provincial government's proposal for the state to oversee health care resources, the profession was defending its relationship to the public as a private transaction, and defining the public as a group of individual patients – patients who, incidentally, could afford doctors' fees. The most adamant supporters of doctors in Saskatchewan during this time were the Keep Our Doctors (KOD) Committees, which were grassroots groups that were started by middle-class housewives, or "anxious mothers," and "common folk" who were afraid that the quality of health care for their families would diminish under state administration. Eventually, professional and business interest groups that were opposed to the health insurance program planned by the CCF government took over this movement.[9] Hence, the medical profession's appeal to the doctor-patient relationship in its argument against the government's proposal had a particular class-based inflection that appealed to the middle and upper classes.

As noted, for the medical profession, the public was a group of private individuals, whose unique health requirements could be met only by an attending physician who was intimately knowledgeable about an individual's life as a whole. By the mid-twentieth century, medical professions across the Western and Westernized worlds, including Canada, adopted the World Health Organization's definition of health as "a state of complete physical, mental and social well-being, and not merely the absence of disease or infirmity."[10] The Canadian medical profession maintained that social aspects of health remained an individual issue, because health status varied according to the unique physiological, genetic, and social makeup of individuals. Noted one Canadian doctor, "It should be made very clear that even the definition of what constitutes health is an individual decision which varies tremendously."[11] In this model, all affairs of health, including illness prevention, diagnosis, and treatment, took place as an individualized interaction between a doctor and a patient. As another physician wrote, the "doctor-patient relationship is an individual activity. While it is true today that there is often a third party in the form of prepaid scheme, yet this third party does not play any part in the spiritual and professional relationship between doctor and patient."[12] This describes a relationship that transcends monetary transaction. It is a sacred relationship that goes beyond economic exchange or a rendering of a service. The physician is bound by an ethical obligation to do no harm, to exercise benevolence, and to observe privacy and confidentiality. For the state to intervene in this relationship was, therefore, to interfere with this sacred and ancient contract between a person and an attending physician. To extend this rationale, doctors were obligated to stand up against the state on behalf of their patients to preserve the sanctity of this private relationship.

Meanwhile, the CCF government argued that health was a fundamental human right, which was to be protected and ensured by the state, along with other social supports and services. The Great Depression had spurred various levels of government across Canada, particularly on the Prairies, which were disproportionately affected by plunging wheat prices, to implement a range of state-funded social services in order to respond to dire poverty among the predominantly agricultural and rural population. Well before the Great Depression there were union hospitals, which were municipally run facilities that paid doctors through tax revenue. The union hospitals began in Sarnia, Saskatchewan, in 1914 and had increased in number to thirty-two across the province by 1930.[13] These hospitals were the predecessor of cooperatively run community clinics that employed doctors on a salary basis,[14] and these clinics, in turn, became the foundation of the CCF government's model for a tax-funded and state-administered health insurance scheme. Thus, for the CCF, health was already an object of statecraft, and a health care–related bureaucracy was already in place to further expand the public health care model across the province. For the government, the public was the citizenry of a welfare state, the blueprint of which had been written during and after the Great Depression. This public had a right to services, including health care, and the state had demonstrated the ability to support this right by administering union hospitals and community clinics. Within this framework, for the medical profession to oppose the arrangement for a tax-funded and state-administered health insurance system was to violate the rights of the public.

The two sides of this health care debate defined health differently, in ways that reinforced their claims to be the protector of the public's health and therefore the body that could best act on behalf of the public interest when it came to health insurance. Hence, the struggle over the terms of the Medical Care Act was simultaneously a battle for the economic and political control over health insurance and the power to shape the discourse of health. The medical profession sought to define health in terms of the doctor-patient relationship, based on the patronage of middle- and upper-class patients, who provided doctors not only with lucrative income streams but also status and prestige. By contrast, a rights-based definition of health fit neatly into the CCF government's welfare governance perspective, which had been the foundation of party's successful electoral strategy.[15]

Medicine and Statecraft

Although representatives of the medical profession and the provincial government sat across from each other at the bargaining table, engaging in heated arguments about health insurance, these two groups had not always been entirely at odds with one another, historically speaking. Medicine and statecraft had become closely integrated in the early part of the twentieth century. Public hospitals provided poorer citizens with access to health care while providing doctors with a livelihood as well as test subjects for clinical studies. During the Great Depression, the Saskatchewan government provided capital grants to new hospitals in rural areas and even paid individual doctors' salaries through hospitals, rehabilitation centres, inmate health in prisons, and geriatric centres, well before the debates about the Medical Care Act in the 1950s and early 1960s.[16] This type of government-funded infrastructure provided the field with training grounds for medical residents and laboratories for biomedical research, allowing medicine to further develop its scientific research and increasingly complex fields of specialization. Robin F. Badgley and Samuel Wolfe, who wrote extensively about the events in Saskatchewan during this time, observed that "the doctors acted like nineteenth century laissez-faire private entrepreneurs in economic affairs, while spending a large portion of their lives applying the technology ... in publicly owned workshops."[17]

Public funds and infrastructure provided medicine with the means to retreat further into the ivory tower, so that "good medicine" became increasingly associated with bench science, specialization, and long years in medical training and research. Medical disinterestedness in the early twentieth century became synonymous with scientific excellence, but at the price of becoming increasingly enmeshed in state bureaucracy. The medical profession and the provincial state mutually benefited from aligning their resources with one another: doctors had guaranteed income during economic depression and access to state-funded clinics and resources, and the provincial government had a new object of statecraft – the health of the citizenry. The standoff over the Medical Care Act was thus the culmination of a gradual historical process by which the state and the medical profession came together during a period of economic crisis under a common interest – that is, the health of the population – to then find themselves vying for control over this shared interest when the immediate crisis subsided.

The alignment of medicine and the state is reminiscent of Michel Foucault's extensive work on statecraft and other forms of expert knowledge production. In *The Birth of Biopolitics*, Foucault describes how a new form of governing rationale emerged with the rise of European nation states after the decline of the monarchy. This art of government, or "governmentality," was not based on the might of the prince to take or spare life, but rather on the interest of the state to maintain itself for its own sake. The concept of biopolitics was Foucault's attempt to write against an ideology-based framing of the state as an institution of coercion or allowances, and instead to draw on his historical analysis and suggest that the modern state is legible only in the practices through which it seeks to know, understand, classify, and track its population for the purpose of maintaining itself – in other words, the politics of life. The health of the population was an area in which a complex network of knowledge, practices, professions, and institutions emerged and were enrolled in the state project to minimize disease and illness, maximize the output of the workforce, and manage the population from birth to death. The clash between the medical profession and the CCF government in Saskatchewan shows that the enrolment of medical experts in the state project to manage the health of the population was neither obvious nor straightforward. During this time, which is prior to the introduction of the economic logic that is often called neo-liberalization to health care policy and administration, we see a strong antagonism from the medical profession, a key expert group in the health care system, to the idea of becoming integrated into the state apparatus, yet all the while benefiting from state resources.

In addition to arguing for the sanctity of the doctor-patient relationship as a private contract, the Saskatchewan medical profession also highlighted its medical expertise as the grounds for the profession's authority to decide matters of payment. Similar to the public health discourse of the nineteenth century, the profession in the mid-twentieth century argued that its expert knowledge extended to determining how the health of the population would be administered. Said an editorial in the *Canadian Medical Association Journal* (*CMAJ*): "The monstrous nonsense that 'health is too important to be entrusted to doctors' should be scotched. The task ahead, that of providing more abundant and more equitably distributed health services, can only be assumed by professional people working in free collaboration with responsible citizens from every level in the community."[18] The profession called for an independent commission, which included representatives from the profession, to oversee the administration of health care planning, while the government wanted an organization composed of elected members under the provincial public health department.[19] The profession also sought to discredit the CCF government by claiming that politics was not the legitimate space in which to contemplate health insurance. As a contributor to the *CMAJ* remarked, "I lack supreme confidence in the infinite wisdom of government in [health services] or other highly technical fields."[20] The medical profession sought to frame health insurance as primarily a medical issue and to position doctors as the only experts who could legitimately speak about it. Meanwhile, the government pushed back, maintaining that health insurance was a matter for the state: doctors could take part in its planning merely as consultants but could not contribute to decision making at the policy or legislative level.

While, in the nineteenth century, the medical profession successfully claimed that doctors had a moral duty to intervene in matters of public health, by the mid-twentieth century this position became problematic. First, the profession had initially supported state-funded health insurance system in Saskatchewan during the 1940s, when the province's economy was still weak and patients could not pay their medical bills but began to resist it when the economy recovered in the 1950s.[21] Second, by 1959 there were two physician-sponsored private medical insurance companies that covered about one-third of the provincial population.[22] It was difficult for the medical profession to claim a disinterested position without incurring suspicion of having self-interested motivations. Even some doctors expressed uneasiness about meddling in matters of insurance, including one writer to the *CMAJ:* "It is not enough to say that those insuring bodies which originated with the blessing of organized medicine are different and therefore acceptable because they are controlled by the profession. They are in truth controlled by the contingencies of business competition, and medical control, though present, is largely nominal."[23] The medical profession made financial moves in the mid-twentieth century that brought it uncomfortably close to matters of business and economics, both of which are antithetical to the profession's disinterested claim to neutrality and moral integrity, as established in the nineteenth century.

As a last resort, the medical profession tried to portray the CCF government as oppressive and dictatorial, drawing on the prevailing postwar suspicion of communism and fascism. It argued that, should the legislation pass, doctors would become mere employees of a dictatorial state and therefore unable to freely exercise their scientific expertise and medical judgment to ensure quality of care in the spirit of the medical disinterestedness that currently governed them: "The medical profession in Saskatchewan will, to a critical extent, cease to be a profession any longer. It will become a group of doctors under political direction."[24] By extension, the profession framed the proposal for state-administered health insurance as "involuntary servitude" and "civil conscription"[25] of the medical profession by the state. These metaphors conflated the medical imperative to act on behalf of the public interest with the notion that doctors should be free and autonomous from state intervention, drawing on the available anti-communist discourses in North America.

The profession resisted calling the walkout on 1 July 1962 a strike, but, regardless, withdrawing medical services was perceived by the public as a violation of medicine's ethical obligation to do no harm.[26] The profession insisted that the government's position on health insurance constituted an "inescapable dilemma" in response to which it had no choice but to walk out, but not before physicians "placated [their] individual and collective conscience by establishing a safe emergency medical service to look after the essential needs of the Saskatchewan people."[27] Until the walkout, the Saskatchewan medical profession was under the impression that it had the public's support, due to the high-profile activities of the Keep Our Doctors Committees and the partisan press in the province, which vilified the CCF government and supported the medical profession's efforts to bar the Medical Care Act.[28] But the profession misread the national press to its own detriment – when the news of the walkout hit the papers outside the province, the profession was taken off guard by the onslaught of criticisms.[29]

The ultimate version of the act that was agreed upon by both the profession and the government was a compromise solution that retained the doctor-patient model through a voluntary fee-for-service system. At the same time, the act enabled the state to control the administrative side of universal care. Thus, the legislative structure supported hybrid notions of health and the public in terms of both individualized and collective models.[30]

The standoff between the medical profession and the provincial government in Saskatchewan shows that the enrolment of medicine as an extension of statecraft was neither straightforward nor even. Indeed, similar events unfolded in 1986, twenty-four years after the doctors' strike in Saskatchewan, when Ontario doctors went on strike in protest of the proposed Bill 94, which would have impeded extra billing by doctors in Ontario. With respect to the Ontario strike, Eric M. Meslin argues that doctors hold an untenable ethical position in a state-funded health care system: they are bound at the same time to their moral obligation toward patients and the public (autonomy of patients) on the one hand and to economic obligations toward their profession and those who rely on them for their livelihood (autonomy of self and the profession) on the other.[31] The same tensions were at play during the 1960s in Saskatchewan. While the medical profession during the latter period tried to merge the two moral obligations under a single discourse of medical disinterestedness, it was unsuccessful and lost the faith of the public. Ontario doctors faced similar outcomes in 1986 when Bill 94 was ultimately passed and the medical profession struggled to salvage its damaged reputation in the eyes of the public in the aftermath of the strike.

Early twentieth-century medicine benefited from state infrastructures but resisted becoming an arm of the state. With the proposal for a state-administered health insurance system by the Saskatchewan government, the medical profession found itself in an arena with an elected government that had a popular platform of welfare governance and with the national media, whose opinions on the matter the profession had misread. The medical profession failed to extend its authority in health and illness to health insurance and, by the extension, to the political field. This failure brought with it the alarming realization for organized medicine that the scientific expertise of doctors could not guarantee the autonomy of medicine as a field. This realization prompted professional medicine to reflect on what it meant to be disinterested in ways that were sympathetic to the needs of the public, whose faith the profession had lost. A new set of discourses and strategies emerged to repair the profession's relationship with the public and to reinvigorate its claim to medical disinterestedness.

Turning "the Social" into a Medical Concept

Although the medical profession was surprised by the national press's negative reactions to the doctors' walkout in Saskatchewan, it was no surprise that for years the profession had been losing touch with the public, on whose behalf it claimed to act. In the nineteenth century, professional medicine merged scientificness (defined as learned rationality) and morality (defined in terms of gentlemanliness) into a cohesive discourse of medical disinterestedness. In the twentieth century, however, the harmony between science and morality went askew. Science, fuelled by innovations in microbiology, pharmacological, and surgical technologies, the emergence of new medical specialties, and an increased emphasis on medical research, became detached from the moral and ethical preoccupations of medicine. In the years leading up to, during, and after the Saskatchewan affair, doctors began to wonder whether medicine's tunnel-visioned search for scientific knowledge had created a perception of the medical profession as disconnected from the interest of the public: "Society is interested in the social and economic aspects of medicine. Doctors tend to withdraw from such strange things into the safety of 17-ketosteroid estimations."[32] Some physicians began to portray too great a focus on science as a self-indulgence that led medicine astray from its moral responsibilities to the public: "If medicine wants to withdraw into itself and become an esoteric and specialized science, such as atomic physics, the profession will become a follower of public opinion, not its architect, an employee of the public, not a servant of the people."[33] Indeed, doctors began to suspect that an overemphasis on science was detrimental to the ideal of medical disinterestedness on the whole: "*Idolatry*: Here the golden calf is science. Many of us have apparently come to worship it, convinced that it alone is medical science and that when all the rituals of scientific protocol have been observed, the patient has been treated fully and well."[34] When the doctors' walk-out in Saskatchewan drew a lacklustre crowd of supporters and much condemnation from the press, it was clear that the profession had lost the faith of the public, without which medical disinterestedness has no meaning. As one writer in the *CMAJ* put it, "We have, of ourselves, no right to practice medicine. It is a privilege granted by each one of our patients."[35] The loss of the public's faith in the medical profession spurred a change in the way organized medicine saw itself, its priorities, and its raison d'être.

Many in the medical profession called for a more socially attuned and more humane form of medicine to repair the profession's credibility in the eyes of the public. Medical periodicals paid heightened attention to issues and topics that were outside of what was strictly "medical." For example, the *CMAJ* published discussions of the possibility of physicians working with social scientists "so that the social origins and consequences of disease may be studied and counteracted more effectively."[36] Some observed that "no longer does the doctor contend unavailingly with numbers of communicable diseases," but "rather, he is faced with complex problems of an aging population, accidents and industrial disease, mental illness and many others."[37] Some went so far as to point to the "distortions which are thrust upon us from the advertising market" and that could lead to "medical matters of social importance" such as suicide, hysteria, and illusory ideas.[38] Contributors to the *CMAJ* expressed concerns about the representations of health and illness in the mass media, where "doctors are not very effective in presenting their views to the public," noting that, "as a profession we have a responsibility when it comes apparent that the public is not being adequately informed on matters of significance" and when "the coverage of events, which in important respects are medical, is unsatisfactory."[39] One contributor reminded his colleagues that medicine was originally "the social science with a dynamic concept and with knowledge" before it became "a conservative self-restrictive profession instead of a widely based social science constantly broadening its scope."[40] Family physicians began to include "a wide range of non-medical activities" among their professional roles and to argue that "the good family doctor is able to deal with most of the ills of people, and knows when and where to get help for the remainder."[41]

Such statements demonstrate a mixture of ideas that question the limits and range of medicine and its rightful domain. What is science and what is non-science? What is medicine and what is non-medicine? Did medicine need to start rethinking its scope of knowledge and practice, or did it simply need to start including domains of knowledge and practice that were once considered to be the non-medical and non-scientific? Out of these concerns, a concept began to gain traction and increasing solidity, a concept that I call "the social" – a category of discourse that refers to moral concerns of medicine at this time, in particular the question of what it means for doctors as individuals and as a professional group to be socially attuned to individual patients and to the public at large. Questions about the relationship between science and medicine and between medicine and the social unfolded mainly in the domains of public health and general practice, two medical disciplines that had been in decline because of their perceived lack of scientificness in an era of specialization and technical innovation.

Public health, which had played a pivotal role in establishing medical disinterestedness in the nineteenth century, was, by the mid-twentieth century, on the bottom rungs of the hierarchy of medical specialties and faced the threat of being ousted from the medical curriculum.[42] The shift toward scientization and specialization in medicine had coincided with what S.E.D. Shortt describes as the golden age of general practice and its sudden demise. The expansion of scientific medicine brought unprecedented legitimacy for generalist physicians, but it also quickly placed them in positions of inferiority compared to their specialized peers.[43] Indeed, by the 1950s, general practice was rumoured to be about to become obsolete, to be replaced by teams of specialists working together in clinical settings.[44] Yet it was precisely the perceived lack of scientificness that made the two disciplines of public health and general practice more humane faces of medicine and ideal spaces within which to work through the problem of re-establishing the moral legitimacy of professional medicine. The goal was not to completely abandon existing scientific ideals of medical research and specialization, but to elevate the status of public health and general practice as respectable specialties. Such a move would re-establish a harmony in medicine between scientific standards and moral obligations in a manner that would be acceptable to both the public and the medical profession. Within these two medical disciplines, the discourse of "the social" became inflected through the emerging scientific discourses of the new social sciences, the result of which was that the notion of the social took shape primarily in terms of individual behaviour and the psychotherapeutic value of the doctor-patient relationship. Professional medicine articulated the social in terms that allowed it to respond to criticisms about its moral integrity and commitment to public good without having to compromise its scientific objectives.

Public Health

By the 1950s, concerted efforts toward medical education reform would save public health from being cut out of the medical curriculum and would encourage teaching the subject in a way that integrated local governmental and voluntary agencies for hands-on learning rather than ivory-tower teaching.[45] Public health, as a branch of medicine that is concerned with the more social aspects of health, such as education and sanitation, presented an existing structural and symbolic framework through which medicine could re-invest its interest in matters of society and "lead the social development of our society."[46] Meanwhile, public health had been developing into an area with a set of knowledge, practices, and agents independent from medicine. In the late nineteenth and the early twentieth century, public health and medicine had converged on the issue of disease prevention and treatment, but the two sides began to diverge significantly after the Second World War. Public health turned to behavioural models of risk at the population level while medicine pursued individualized treatments at the level of the patient.[47] The early twentieth century was also the dawn of mass media and, although there were public health physicians, much of the public education work in preventive health and hygiene was conducted by a new profession of health educators who were not trained in medicine but who were media savvy.

To counter this trend, the medical profession, both domestic and international, worked to position doctors at "the apex of the health education pyramid ... to ensure the scientific accuracy of what is taught." It argued that the goal of public health education was more than the dissemination of information and included "changing attitudes and behaviour,"[48] a task that that it claimed was most suited to the physician, who would be able to command respect and credibility in a way that a health educator could not.[49]

In general, there was a push within the profession toward thinking of the social responsibility of medicine in terms of an emphasis on human behaviour pertaining to public health: "An enlightened attitude towards human behaviour may pay bigger research dividends than an electron microscope."[50] Yet the reality was that doctors were not experts on such behavioural matters. However, in the area of the social, some doctors were willing to acknowledge the expertise of social scientists, who had developed their craft into a credible science, which included tracking and quantifying individual social behaviours.[51] The sudden mention of social scientists in the *CMAJ* during this moment and the debates about whether they could be seen as colleagues or consultants in matters of public health, or could be ignored altogether as ultimately not disinterested,[52] demonstrate the degree to which doctors felt insecure about their lack of legitimate expertise in social matters.

Professional medicine's interest in the social emerged at the juncture of two approaches in public health – preventive medicine and social medicine – which were grounded in quite different sets of epistemological and political tenets. Preventive medicine continued and built on older public health practices related to sanitation, public works, and vaccination and was concerned with preventing the spread of disease and illness, which by the mid-twentieth century predominantly meant addressing chronic illnesses rather than communicable diseases.[53] By involving itself in health education, professional medicine could "indicate [to the public] that the medical profession has a genuine interest in preventive medicine in addition to its interest in 'prophylactic medicine.'"[54]

Meanwhile, social medicine emerged through various late nineteenth-century social reform movements that positioned medicine in the arena of social policy and social movements. Dorothy Porter argues that, in Latin America, social medicine became detached from academic disciplines and interlinked with Marxism-inspired political movements, resulting in an attention to structural issues of health, such as access to medicine. In contrast, in Anglo-America, particularly in the United States, social medicine struggled to maintain its disciplinary status, and in the process was influenced by medicine's biomedical and therapeutic approaches. There were pockets of grassroots social medicine efforts in the United States, including the development of community health clinics for and by African Americans during the civil rights movement,[55] but, on the whole, Anglo-American social medicine adopted a more behaviourist model focusing on individualized lifestyles and risk factors for chronic illnesses.[56]

The Anglo-American version of social medicine was at the basis of the Department of Social and Behavioural Medicine at the University of Saskatchewan, which was established in 1959–60. Its first department head, Alexander Robertson, wrote several articles in the *CMAJ* in order to promote his department's vision of public health, which he saw as different from preventive medicine: "I just happen to think that 'social' embraces the totality of what we are trying to achieve more successfully than 'preventive.'"[57] The department combined the traditional tenets of public health, such as sanitation, with new epidemiological approaches to chronic illnesses based on morbidity and mortality measures, health administration, and social aspects of disease. Robertson explained that the social aspects of disease were "where many would say that the art of medicine and the science of medicine overlap,"[58] an area that was increasingly examined by sociologists, whose attention to "the study of social forces, social change and social groups ... can help medicine unravel the eternally fascinating riddles of cause and effect."[59] By elevating the status of the sociologist to that of a scientific colleague, public health medicine sought to bring social expertise into medicine's realm and to present medicine as a discipline and doctors as a profession as genuinely interested in society.

However, only specific social science perspectives were welcomed and invoked, specifically, those that focused on the individual "man in his social state" as an atomized subject with a linear causal relationship to their environment, or, as Robertson put it, "the implications of the health state of an individual upon his social environment, and the role of his social environment in determining his state of health."[60] For Robertson, the sociologist colleague could help medicine think about social factors to help bridge the domain of medicine and the domain of the social, or to "play a part in reconciling the apparently divergent trends of modern medicine, the conflict between the scientist and the humanist in all of us." The sociologist's role was primarily that of a translator, exercising their ability to "use language intelligible to a layman to explain his concepts" and to "at least begin to apply quantitative measurements to social phenomena."[61] Social science was allowed to be part of medicine if it could fit into medicine's existing models that focused on individual patients and their behaviours, and if it could assist medicine by making the social legible for the profession, which in this case meant quantitative and deductive analyses. This view of the social stands in contrast with imagining medicine's role in social policy more broadly. Behavioural models from the social sciences provided an easy framework for medicine to become more socially attuned, and therefore more morally responsible toward the public, all the while maintaining existing standards of what counted as legitimate scientific knowledge in medicine.

General Practice

At the same time that public health rose to the centre of attention for the medical profession in its goal to align its ongoing scientific objectives with the new concern to be more socially attuned and moral, general practice also emerged as a high priority for the profession. During the Saskatchewan affair, doctors claimed that the state's intervention in health care threatened the sanctity of the doctor-patient relationship, but the practice of medicine had been veering away from this model for some time. General practice and the family physician, the corner-stones of traditional medical practice, had been in a steady decline. Fewer doctors chose to become family physicians, as more and more extended their education in order to specialize or to conduct medical research.[62] The critique of the medical profession as elitist highlighted a vast distance between the profession and the public, and many in the profession saw general practice as an already existing way to bridge this distance. General practitioners emphasized their intimate involvement with patients and their affairs at various stages in their lives. Despite the increasing complexities of medical treatments, they claimed people still "like to know their doctor," who "has always been, and will again be, a rock standing safe in the shifting sands of urban social change."[63] Indeed, it was often stated by physicians writing in medical journals during this time that while the medical profession had lost the public's faith, the individual physician, particularly the family doctor, still commanded a lot of respect and trust from his or her patients: "Let's face the fact that in the eyes of our sickly patients we may be demigods; in the eyes of the collective public we seem to be a group of monopolistic money-grubbers, bloated with self-importance, intolerant of intrusion in to our private domain and martyred in pseudo-sacrificial devotion to our indigent brethren."[64] While a specialist might have mastery over a highly technical aspect of medicine, the general practitioner claimed a better knowledge of the patient as a person by adopting a holistic approach to care, paying attention to "non-medical activities" as well as the patient's social and economic environment.[65] General practitioners overcame their lack of specialization by highlighting their rapport with patients, which allowed them to carve out a role for themselves as trusted mediators between esoteric medical knowledge and patients. They positioned themselves as someone "who will guide [patients] through the maze of medical technology, and who will provide genuine interest and friendship which means so much more than techniques."[66] General practitioners' claim to their specialty took on a gendered discourse that framed the existing trend toward clinical and esoteric medicine in masculine terms, such as "aggressive and scientific,"[67] while their own practices were more feminine, enmeshed in the personal and domestic life of patients. General practice provided a way to think about establishing rapport with the public in terms of individualized relationships with patients, which was in keeping with the profession's position that health was an individual matter.

Despite their emphasis on the importance of emotional and social aspects of patient care, general practitioners still had to contend with the yardstick of science that dominated medicine. Thus, they avoided a nostalgia for the nineteenth-century golden age of the family doctor who travelled by "horse and buggy" to visit patients.[68] Instead, they reinvented themselves in the age of specialization and scientific medicine as a legitimate sub-specialty grounded in scientific excellence. The College of General Practice was established in 1954 in order to organize and oversee a more comprehensive education in family medicine as a specialty,[69] and general practitioners were encouraged to teach at medical schools in order to train more of their own.[70] The newly formed college developed fellowships on specialized medical topics, such as palliative care and geriatrics, in order to augment the scientific status of general practice through certification and continued education that emulated the specialization model.[71] General practitioners also argued that the size of their clinical practices made it easier to conduct research on diseases and illnesses that could not be found or tracked well in hospitals, such as chronic diseases and illnesses related to age or heredity.[72]

Along with organizational changes to elevate general practice as a specialty, there was a move to reinterpret and update the value of the doctor-patient encounter in the context of the increasing incidence of psychiatric disorders. While some claimed that a continuing emphasis on the doctor-patient relationship portrayed the medical profession as archaic,[73] others highlighted this relationship as "the art of medicine" or "bedside medicine" and asserted that the profession should pay attention to such matters, given that "disease forms themselves have changed" from the "gross organic lesions" of the early part of the twentieth century to "the psychoses" that in the mid-twentieth century "fill half the total number of hospital beds."[74] Thus, general practice teamed up with another lowly medical specialty – psychiatry – that was just gaining momentum at the time with developments in psychopharmaceuticals (such as tranquilizers),[75] a move toward more humane methods of psychotherapy,[76] and new categories of psychiatric conditions with the publication of the first edition of the *Diagnostic and Statistical Manual of Mental Disorders* in 1952.[77] This new and more humane psychiatry provided scientific credibility to what general practitioners had been doing simply by virtue of being family physicians: listening to patients speak, providing them with assurance, and noting the ways in which their social, emotional, and financial lives affected their health – all of which the discourse of psychiatry rearticulated as "the therapeutic significance of the medical interview"[78] – and "helping people to solve the emotional and social problems created by crises at various periods of life"[79] as part of "the science of man as a thinking, dreaming, socializing and uniquely human being."[80] Psychiatry, therefore, transformed what was considered to be the art of medicine into a viable therapeutic methodology, thereby raising the status of the general practitioner to the ranks of specialists and researchers. Psychiatry, too, gained status by linking itself with general practice, which provided ideal clinical access to everyday patients for psychiatric conditions – the social diseases of modern urban life – that were fast becoming the predominant health concern for general practice.[81] Hence, general practice and psychiatry entered into a mutually beneficial arrangement, reinforcing one another's scientific credibility. In the process, general practice embraced a particular notion of the social, that of a therapeutic encounter between an individual doctor and an individual patient or family unit.

***

Doctors took seriously the years of mounting criticisms that they were elitist professionals who were more concerned about their own political and economic power and what was under the microscope than with the plight of their patients or the public. Doctors came to see that their scientific standards had overshadowed their moral obligations, to the point that they could not sufficiently convince the public or themselves of their disinterestedness. The notion of "the social" emerged as a pressing issue. Public health medicine and general practice, two disciplines facing rapid decline during the height of scientific medicine, became ideal venues through which doctors as a group could regain their credibility as socially attuned and humane experts who were deserving of the public's trust. The developments in these two disciplines toward more behaviourist and psychiatric approaches presented methods and therapeutic categories that aligned with existing scientific standards in medicine. As public health medicine and general practice rose in the ranks of medical hierarchy, the two disciplines shed some of their "art" in order to gain credibility among other specialties. Public health medicine increasingly focused on individualized notions of social behaviour, and general practice rearticulated the doctor-patient relationship in the psychiatric terms of psychotherapy.[82]

Public Relations and Media Work

In addition to turning inward to reflect on what medicine is and should be, as a way to win back public trust, doctors as individuals and as a profession also turned their gaze outward to an area that they had hitherto renounced: public relations and media. During the years of tension with the CCF government in Saskatchewan, the Canadian Medical Association had provided public relations packages to doctors to help persuade their patients and the public of the validity of their position in the political debate.[83] However, doctors found it challenging to accept the idea of engaging in public relations or talking to the media, tactics associated with politics and the business world, as legitimately medical and disinterested. It took considerable discursive work to convince them that media work was an appropriate solution to the problem of the profession's relationship to the public, and one that was in line with medical disinterestedness.

The medical profession was already doing public relations and media work in the mid-twentieth century. In the 1950s, the *CMAJ* published an American survey of public attitudes toward doctors, which found that the public's negative opinion toward doctors stemmed primarily from long waits in waiting rooms, inattentiveness by doctors, and unfair medical charges.[84] Around the same time, the *CMAJ* produced a series of editorial columns called "Public Relations Forum," published from 1955 to 1956, which offered doctors strategies to improve their relationship with patients and the public, ranging from how to train the receptionist at one's private practice to how to talk to the press.[85] The Canadian Medical Association (CMA) highlighted the state of the doctor-public relationship as a pressing medical problem that had to be addressed through better lines of communication with the public. The chairman of the CMA's Committee on Public Relations defended his work by invoking the association's original objectives from 1867, including "to direct and control public opinion in regard to the duties and responsibility of medical men," arguing that "all modern techniques and lines of communication must be used" in order to be faithful to this objective.[86] He concluded that doctors have "a collective responsibility to present the profession's actions and views in a light which will enhance our reputation in the eyes of our fellow citizens,"[87] echoing the nineteenth-century discourse that connected obligation to the profession with obligations to the public. The CMA framed public relations as a remedy for the unfavourable public image of the medical profession, which doctors as a group perceived to be caused by the public's misunderstanding of the true intentions of the profession. In the context of the medical insurance debate in Saskatchewan, the associated noted the importance of convincing the public that its opposition to the government's proposal was not based on a self-interested desire to protect doctors' lucrative incomes but rather to ensure better quality of care for all: "For while the public would have supported us in resisting such restrictions of our liberty as would have brought about a deterioration of our service to them, they were entirely without sympathy with any effort on our part to resist a threat to our income."[88]

Public relations as a professional field emerged at the beginning of the twentieth century as a strategy to harmonize the relationship between diverse fields such as government and politics, business and commerce, and the democratic notion of a public with rights, including entitlements to transparent governance and business practices.[89] After the Second World War, however, public relations tended to evoke memories of Nazi propaganda and, at the same time, became increasingly connected to advertising and marketing, all of which were associated with manipulation. Indeed, the chairman of the CMA's Committee on Public Relations noted that "it is quite apparent that there are some people who associate a medical public relations program with that of advertising or high-pressured publicity."[90] It was one thing to have doctors agree that the public image of medicine was a problem, but quite another to convince them that public relations was a legitimate solution. To turn to a business and political method that was widely associated with deception would be to confirm the public's accusations that doctors were motivated by financial gain rather than by the common good. The CMA and the *Canadian Medical Association Journal* did considerable discursive work to convince its readership that public relations was a legitimate medical practice that was in line with the tenets of medical disinterestedness. In the process, they deployed advertising and public relations strategies on doctors. Advertising is based on shaping the values and connotations associated with a product, reframing and recontextualizing that product so that its original meaning morphs into something that is appealing and novel and instills desire for consumption.[91] Public relations directs this advertising strategy in order to associate particular – usually positive – meanings and values with a person or a group. Often, this process involves using euphemisms to rhetorically reframe what are normally perceived as negative traits into positive ones, or to rearticulate neutral qualities into more explicitly appealing ones.[92] Finally, public relations strategies continuously project this revised representation of the person or group so that it becomes its new image.

The CMA and the *CMAJ* sought to dissociate public relations from the world of politics, commerce, and advertising, where it was a strategy of manipulation, and instead to convince doctors that public relations was a legitimate professional practice of disinterested medicine. The CMA and the *CMAJ* claimed that public relations were a means of creating a more effective line of communication with the public to "inform and persuade," with the intention of establishing "good public relationships – good will and harmony."[93] The chairman of the Committee of Public Relations differentiated between "good public relations" and "the promotional methods frequently used by those who oppose ethical medical practice" and with whom doctors "are in competition." "Good public relations" was not about deception but merely stating the truth as it was. It could "interpret intelligently the viewpoint of orthodox medicine in Canada" using "high standards" that were "directed and approved by doctors who are members of the Standing Committee on Public Relations."[94] Another editorial on public relations compared it with the public health strategy of preventive medicine: "the practice of public relations, like that of medicine, should emphasize prevention, preserving the health of public attitude by precluding any sources of misunderstanding or conflict.[95] The aim of such a preventive approach was for the profession to "[reveal] itself as being interested in the welfare of the community and its citizens" and to "[tell] the public, within the bounds of good ethics, of course, about one's community spirit."[96] In other words, the intention was not to deceive or to manipulate people into believing something that was false, but to better convey what was already an established truth – that is, doctors' honourable intentions.

As the issue of payment was discussed more and more in relation to the health insurance debate, the discursive strategies of public relations provided a way for doctors to navigate the uncomfortable and problematic situations where they negotiated payment with patients. Through euphemism, doctors could transform their conversations with patients about money from a necessary evil to good medical practice: "It is not too mercenary to help a patient budget for his medical care" because doctors can "smooth the way and relieve the patient's uncertainty" by openly discussing the issue of payment.[97] This strategy required doctors to see that their role included an understanding of and a sensitivity to patients' financial situations, so that they were able to convince reluctant patients both to accept "the doctor's moral right to charge a fee and [to] consider the cost of medicine as a desirable 'investment.'"[98] Presenting fees as an investment highlighted the connection between payment and care and made the former seem reasonable and more palatable. Such efforts to transform public perception first required that doctors see that their practice as doctors included the work of transforming the negative public opinion of the profession into a positive one, even if it meant that doctors saw this part of their practice as being not so different from the work of public relations agents. The onus was on the doctor: "All the public relations programs in the world cannot remove the doctor's responsibilities for paying attention to the improvement of doctor-patient relationships."[99] Indeed, "it is in [the individual doctor's] daily contact with people, in the office, in the club, on the golf course, in church, wherever it may be, that he must launch his attack against poor public relationships."[100]

However, the scientific ideals still dominated medicine, and the idea that doctors could be confused with a smooth-talking publicist, an advertising agent, or even a well-meaning financial adviser was a lot for some members of the profession to stomach. For doctors to be skilled in self-promotion and in shaping the perception of the public required that they acquire the dispositions and know-how associated with the economic and political world, which would in turn mean that they did not possess a disinterested habitus. Moreover, as some writers observed, such talents ran counter to those required in the traditional practice of medicine: "We ... are not experts in speech making, or the art of public relations. Least of all are we experts in politics. A good doctor wants only to practice good medicine."[101] Also, there was a widespread understanding among doctors that individual doctors, particularly family physicians, were still held in high regard; thus, many rejected the proposition that the public image of the profession was a legitimately medical problem. Those who raised the alarm about public perception of the profession emphasized the responsibility of doctors toward the professional group to "enhance our reputation in the eyes of our fellow citizens"[102] in order to secure their position of leadership in matters of health and illness. Yet the growing unpopularity of the medical profession compelled many doctors to take a more cautious stance in the name of humility and to avoid taking such authoritative leadership roles for granted. Some doctors argued that "the reputation of the physician must be based on his integrity and knowledge and not on what the patient will say, or on the reaction of an public body."[103] Doctors, they maintained, did not need to be so conscious of the perception of the public in the first place because medical authority stemmed from the wisdom and maturity of experts who remained distant from the lowly affairs of the public, who did not understand what doctors did. Doctors simply had to demonstrate their honourable intentions toward the public by relying on the existing high standards of care – science would speak for itself because "neither the doctor's work nor the doctor-patient relationship needs explaining. It cannot be explained. It is based on faith."[104]

The adverse response to the walkout on 1 July 1962 produced a new attitude among doctors, as they came to attribute their failure to win public support in their struggle against the provincial government to an ineffective public relations strategy: "the public image, presence and voice, broadcast by the representatives of the medical organization of Saskatchewan was far weaker, more uncertain, clumsier and far less articulate than that of the confident, cocky and misleading representatives of the other side."[105] Those who took this position argued that, had doctors in the province and the nation as a whole taken their public image more seriously, they could have avoided being misunderstood by the public, and the public being misled by the government.[106] Specifically, contributors to the *CMAJ* after the Saskatchewan affair claimed that "freedom was the issue, not money,"[107] and further argued that "the public would have supported [the province's doctors] in resisting such restrictions of [their] liberty"[108] because "most of the best types of men who would be motivated to enter a noble and free profession would no longer be so motivated if their future is to be servility in an undesirable form of civil service,"[109] a result that would ultimately harm the public. Although doctors accused the provincial government of conducting "very effective propaganda,"[110] many admonished the CMA for "the appalling[ly] poor job of public relations"[111] that presented an "inept and confused picture."[112] They criticized the association for relying on the scientific merits of medicine, noting that such a strategy that was based on naïveté rather than maturity, on "false pride" rather than honour, and on the "false assumption that honesty and dedication to humanity will of necessity shine through and cast a true image; and that nobody would cheat such a naively honest and devoted man as the doctor."[113] In adopting such a strategy, they asserted, the profession had done a great disservice to the public by not protecting them from government propaganda.

The idea that public relations on the part of the medical profession could or should be part of a service to the public to convey accurate information fell neatly into doctors' concerns about the role of the media in public health education. They saw such education as pandering to the public's demand for entertainment – for example, showing shocking surgical procedures on live television, rendering medicine into a spectacle[114] – rather than presenting legitimate information on health. However, structural barriers prevented individual doctors from communicating directly with the public. The code of ethics of the CMA explicitly forbade doctors, except those in designated roles in executive positions on the CMA, to talk to the public on medical matters: "All opinions on medical subjects which are communicated to the laity by any medium, whether it be a public meeting, the lay press, radio or television should be presented as from some organized and recognized medical society or association and not from an individual physician."[115]

This part of the code originated from earlier concerns at the turn of the twentieth century by the profession about doctors who advertised their private practices and personal concoctions. By mid-century, such types of advertising were antiquated, as medications were no longer produced by individual physicians but by a burgeoning pharmaceutical industry. However, this section of the code lingered into the mid-century and demonstrated a more general feeling of caution among the profession that any practice of self-promotion that was based on the logic of the economic field would be read as unscientific and not disinterested.[116] By framing the issue of communication with the public as a matter of health education and the dissemination of accurate scientific information, however, doctors could bypass the ethical constraints against speaking to the public, and, indeed, could feel obligated to intervene in popular media in the name of promoting scientific truth and providing a public service. In fact, one of the major criticisms by some of members against the CMA after the Saskatchewan affair was the association's conservative position with regard to public relations, which prevented individual doctors from engaging directly with the public, thereby allowing the proliferation of what they claimed was misinformation on health insurance by the CCF government.[117]

As they turned outward from their esoteric worlds of medicine to radio, television, and the press, doctors came up against the field of journalism. William Osler, an influential Canadian physician who revolutionized North American medical education in the early twentieth century, cautioned doctors against the "temptation to toy with the Delilah of the Press," which is "sure to play the harlot, and has left many a man shorn of his strength, namely the confidence of his professional brethren."[118] Echoing Osler's concerns, albeit in less dramatic language, the CMA's code of ethics of 1938 and 1945 stated that "physicians should be extremely cautious in dealing with the Press. A physician should insist, wherever possible, on seeing a proof of what is to be printed under his name or on his authority."[119]

Journalism at the turn of the previous century consisted mainly of the penny press, which was mostly concerned about advertising revenues and relied on sensationalism to sell papers. It was not until the 1920s, following the emergence of public relations industries and government propaganda during the First World War, that the field as a whole began to take the issue of credibility and objectivity seriously, establishing journalism schools and codes of ethics in the name of the public interest.[120] Despite these changes in journalism, there remained fundamental differences in the ways in which science and journalism handled the issue of scientific truth and objectivity. Patrick Champagne and Dominique Marchetti note that science prioritizes established ideas that have been tested extensively to minimize their potential for error, while journalism embraces untested ideas and hypotheses as legitimately objective statements.[121] This argument was evident in the *CMAJ*, which noted that "the practice of medicine is thoughtful, careful and deliberate. It has to be. Newspaper work by the very sense of urgency inherent in it, is almost the opposite to this. It has to be."[122] The deep historical and epistemological differences between the two fields prompted the proposal that doctors had to understand and learn how to navigate the differences. One "Public Relations Forum" column on doctors and the press argued that the problem was not that journalists were not objective or not disinterested enough, but that "much of the misunderstanding stems from the doctor's lack of knowledge of how reporters work."[123] Instead of shunning the press because of these differences, doctors had to become the experts to whom the journalist would turn when reporting on a medical story. Hence, by raising the scientificness and of the field of journalism and the habitus of journalists, doctors sought to justify their dealings with the press.

The public reaction to the doctors' strike in Saskatchewan prompted the medical profession to re-evaluate its emphasis on scientific pursuits and to instead seek to demonstrate social engagement and interest in the public. In the medical profession, the prevailing view was that doctors had failed in the arena of public opinion with regard to the health insurance debate because the public had misunderstood the profession's intentions. To remedy what then became a communication issue, professional medicine embraced public relations and media work – albeit with some hesitance, because these were strategies borrowed from the world of politics and business. To temper the discomfort of adopting practices connected to war propaganda and advertising, the medical profession elevated the scientific status of journalism and framed public relations and media work as part of legitimate medical practice. By working with the media, professional medicine would be fulfilling a public service of providing accurate health information (including the "true" intentions of the profession toward the public) in the most effective means possible, while remaining true to its scientific standards.

***

The events of 1962 in Saskatchewan were not just about doctors going on strike to protect their pay, although money played a pivotal role in the question of health insurance in general, and the discourses used in this strike resonated in other strikes, notably the Ontario doctors' strike in 1986. The Saskatchewan affair is significant for its particular historical backdrop and the discursive responses and shifts that took place with respect to the moral and scientific obligations of doctors. The negotiations over the Medical Care Act in Saskatchewan took place at a time when medicine had achieved overall dominance in matters of health and illness after pushing out other health disciplines in the nineteenth century. Twentieth-century developments further increased medicine's scientificness and its ability to offer successful therapeutic interventions. However, these triumphs came at the expense of losing public trust and support, in whose name doctors claimed to do medicine in the first place. The failure of the doctors' strike in Saskatchewan was a wake-up call to the medical profession that its authority and dominance were not to be taken for granted and that it was not sufficient for medicine to simply offer pharmaceutical solutions and surgical miracles to win public trust. Medical disinterestedness requires both scientificness and moral credibility. Not only was the profession in the public's dog house, but there were other players at the table: the state as the administrative arm of health care and, to a lesser extent, journalism as the public's watchdog each were forces to be reckoned with, with their own interests, definitions of health, and disinterested claims to be working for the public good.

The Saskatchewan case is also significant because certain discursive shifts took place with regard to moral and scientific norms as a result of the conflict. Professional medicine came to foreground family practice and public health, medical disciplines that had been fading in the age of specialization, in its attempt to embrace the social aspects of health and illness as a way to regain public trust and salvage its reputation of disinterestedness and benevolence. "The social" in these practices became synonymous with individualized behaviour and psychiatric states, frames that aligned with the existing model of doctor-patient relationships and with the profession's insistence that health was an individual issue. The profession additionally embraced public and media relations, once morally tainted practices associated with propaganda and advertising, as a respectable aspect of profession practice. Observers argued that more effective communication work through public and media relations would have avoided the public misunderstandings of the intentions of the profession during the Saskatchewan affair. Hence, writers in medical journals described a close medicine-media relationship as a way for doctors to become more socially responsible. In attempting to repair its relationship with the public, the medical profession built a bridge between the field of medicine and the media industry, a move that had important implications for medical publishing, as we will see in the next chapter.

The Paradox of Medical Publishing   **4**

In an effort to rebuild its deteriorating relationship with the public, the Canadian medical profession of the mid-twentieth century embraced public relations and media work. In the process, medicine opened itself up to the media industry, with its own sets of rules, norms, and stakes. This opening became a problem in recent years in relation to medical publishing. On 20 February 2006, the top editors of the *Canadian Medical Association Journal* (*CMAJ*) were fired, stirring considerable controversy in national and international medical circles. While this was not the first time that an editor of a medical journal had been fired, it was the first time that the top editors were sacked in the history of the *CMAJ,* and the circumstances in which the dismissals took place made the action a particularly heated topic.

The editor-in-chief, John Hoey, and senior deputy editor, Anne Marie Todkill, had ushered the journal to significant international prestige over the preceding decade. Their dismissal followed high-profile firings in 1999 at two prominent medical journals – the *Journal of the American Medical Association* (*JAMA*)[1] and the *New England Journal of Medicine* (*NEJM*).[2] In 2004, for the first time in the journal's almost hundred-year history, the management of the *CMAJ* was handed over to a private company, Canadian Medical Association Holdings, which also manages pensions for CMA members. The dismissals took place during a time of increasing corporatization of medical journals, which was accompanied by a threat to editorial independence, one of the most cherished principles of not only medical publishing but the intellectual work of science in general.

The new owners merely stated that the journal needed a "fresh approach,"[3] prompting a rally of support for the dismissed editors and claims that the CMA had violated editorial independence. Scientific journals are an integral part of the intellectual life of scientists in their pursuit of science for the sake of science. However, as a form of media, such journals are also subject to the market forces of circulation figures and, quite often, advertising revenues in order to sustain them. Contemporary science relies on the infrastructure of the publishing industry to disseminate knowledge, making it impossible to completely dissociate scientific work from other social worlds. The debates surrounding the dismissal of the editors of the *CMAJ* and the fate of the journal brought this inherent contradiction within medical science into sharp relief.

The argument that science is inherently social, political, and economic is not new in social studies of science. However, scientists and doctors still persist in dissociating "pure" intellectual science from forces understood to be non-scientific or even unscientific. At the heart of medical publishing is a belief that objectivity in medical research is both possible and desirable, even while the criteria for good scientific research and publishing remain elusive. In the debates that followed the dismissals at the *CMAJ*, objectivity was framed primarily in terms of editorial autonomy. Hoey wrote an editorial in the *Lancet* sharply denounced the firings as a "scandal" and the CMA's actions "deeply troubling."[4] The discussion in medical journals framed the breach in editorial autonomy as the violation of fundamental values of medicine and medical professionalism – "scientific objectivity, respect for patients, health promotion, altruism, truth-telling, leadership and benevolence."[5] These values were taken for granted as stable and as transparent to everyone involved in medical journals, whether as writers, editors, readers, or publishers. Yet, as a Saskatchewan specialist stated, "You can either see medical journals as commercial or scientific enterprises ... but perhaps not both."[6] He pointed to the contradictions in medical publishing, where scientific objectivity required continual negotiation, given the ways in which publishing was corporately structured and financed. Others referred to the ways in which physicians' fees were allocated through the provincial governments in Canada to support their argument that "organized medicine is a political and social entity" in a much broader sense.[7]

In this chapter, I read the position taking by the two sides – the dismissed editors and their supporters versus the journal owners and their supporters – as a struggle over what it means to exercise objectivity in medical publishing in a disinterested manner. The violation of editorial autonomy through the *CMAJ* owners' firing of the editors was the tip of the iceberg. The dismissals became an international controversy because they raised potentially delegitimating questions about medical publishing, with its conflicting imperatives to identify and publicize pure science while maintaining business standards. A close reading of the discourse leading up to and surrounding the dismissal showed deep-seated inconsistencies and contradictions with respect to objectivity and ethics in medical publishing. The events surrounding the dismissal raise questions of how and by whom medical knowledge ought to be reported and disseminated. Indeed, they raise questions of what is legitimate medical knowledge in the first place. In the end, scientific objectivity emerges as an elusive and undefined concept, making it possible to make various, and at times conflicting, claims about what it means to be objective and ethical, based on specific interests – in other words, to enact medical disinterestedness.

Scientific versus Journalistic Ethics

The *CMAJ* editors were dismissed shortly after their disagreement with the journal's owners over an investigative news story that was published on 6 December 2005. The owners had tried to withhold the story, basing their argument on the standards of objectivity and ethics in medical research. The editors defended the story with reference to the standards of investigative reporting in journalism. The editorial writings in international medical journals pointed to the investigative news story incident as the cause of the dismissal, but this dispute revealed more deep-seated contradictions between the rules of scientific research and those of journalism that simultaneously govern medical publishing. In particular, the incident revealed medical publishing as an area within medicine that is susceptible to the forces and rules of others field – journalism and the media industry – specifically with regard to the standards of ethics and objectivity.

The incident began when two medical journalists at the *CMAJ*, Laura Eggertson and Barbara Sibbald, discovered that the Canadian Pharmacists Association (CPhA) was advising pharmacists to collect personal information from women seeking an over-the-counter emergency contraceptive commonly known as Plan B. The CPhA's survey stored details of menstrual cycle, methods of birth control, instances of unprotected sex, and reasons for taking the drug along with prescription data. The journalists raised concerns about privacy and barriers to accessing the drug.[8] As part of their investigation, they had taken testimonials from thirteen women across Canada who had purchased Plan B from local pharmacies but did not inform the pharmacists who dispensed the drug that their dispensing practices were under scrutiny. The CPhA got wind of the story from the federal Privacy Commissioner before the issue went to press. The CPhA's executive director confronted the CMA, asking "whether it was true its reporters were conducting covert research, and whether the research was being carried out in an ethical manner."[9] The journal owners "agreed there was cause for concern"[10] and asked the editors to pull the story on the grounds that it was scientific research and had to follow the ethical requirements of biomedical research – in this case, get informed consent from the pharmacists involved in the investigation. The journal owners argued that the story "could be confused with material in the journal's research section, which is separate and must be reviewed by outside experts."[11] Similar to other medical journals such as the *Lancet*, the *CMAJ* prints peer-reviewed articles that follow ethical protocols of human research and also news material of interest to doctors such as editorials by the editorial board, opinion essays and letters to the editor by doctors across Canada, poetry, book reviews, and obituaries. In order to publish the Plan B story, the editors defined the article as legitimate and responsible journalism but not scientific research. This enabled them to get around the question of informed consent (a research concept, not a journalistic one).

In response to the pressure from the journal owners, the story was published without the women's testimonials, which would have served as real-person citations that are valued in investigative reporting. In his editorial of 3 January 2006, Hoey documented the actions of the CMA as a transgression: "The CMA questioned the propriety of our investigation and the boundary between news reporting and scientific research. Our story was not scientific research, however, but legitimate journalism."[12] When the existing Journal Oversight Committee (JOC), which had been established in 2002 to ensure harmonious relations between the CMA and the editorial board, did not respond to his complaint in a timely manner, Hoey appointed an ad hoc JOC to attend to the matter. The ad hoc JOC echoed Hoey's position that the original Plan B story "represented legitimate and ethically responsible journalism,"[13] and argued that the information obtained through the covert method used "could not have been obtained by other means."[14]

The arguments for and against the Plan B story by the journal editors and owners can be situated in the different ways in which biomedical research and journalism view covert research in their respective fields. Journalism has had a more comfortable relationship with the method because covert investigative reporting helped to blow the whistle on corruption among those in authority, such as during the Watergate scandal. Covert methods helped to augment the credibility of journalism as a profession that is responsible for the public's well-being.[15] However, deception and dishonesty are not unilaterally endorsed in journalism as strategic or morally acceptable. Media philosopher Matthew Kieran notes that the responsibility to uncover truths that concern the public may require the journalist to engage in immoral activities, such as deception, but that the ends of investigative journalism do not justify any means. Rather, "certain actions we normally think of as immoral can be, under certain strict conditions, morally justified."[16] The exact circumstances of these conditions are an ongoing the subject of debate within journalism. Those who supported the *CMAJ* editors, including Canadian newspaper journalists who wrote about the incident, did not question whether Eggertson and Sibbald's choice of method was ethically legitimate. Only the president of the Saskatchewan Medical Association contended that, even within the ethical standards of journalism, "the undercover method used cannot be justified" and "cannot reconcile that editorial freedom can legitimately be used to justify this type of practice."[17] The editors and their supporters instead highlighted the potential harm caused by the actions of the CPhA by invoking the journalistic notion of a public responsibility to seek and reveal truth. By extension, the two journalists were whistle-blowers, and their covert method could be judged as ethically justified. It is important to note here that the support for the Plan B story and its authors was support for a particular type of journalistic practice. Historically, medicine has had an uneasy relationship with journalism, as noted by William Osler's warnings cited in the preceding chapter as well as the experience of the Saskatchewan medical profession during the health insurance debates. The type of journalism invoked by the Plan B story authors and the editors of the *CMAJ* was the "pure" journalism of the twentieth century, post-Watergate, not the sensationalism of the penny press.

The journal owners drew on an entirely different notion of ethics – those of biomedical research – to reject the Plan B story. Biomedicine's position on covert research is less ambiguous than that of journalism. After the horrors of Nazi experimentation and other abuses of humans in research, such as the Tuskegee syphilis study in 1932–72 (where African American men in Alabama were deceived into participating in a research study for decades without their knowledge), international and national ethical protocols for human research have suppressed deception as a research method.[18] These abuses damaged the reputation of science as an altruistic pursuit of knowledge and common good. The Nuremburg Code of 1947 and the Declaration of Helsinki in 1964 outlined the ethical principles of research involving human subjects, and these documents were, in part, efforts by biomedicine to restore its reputation as a truly disinterested enterprise. The documents emphasized full disclosure and consent as the ultimate evidence of the ethical integrity of any research involving human subjects.[19] However, the documents were not legally binding, and their general principles were only unevenly, if at all, integrated into the laws of various states.

The work of biomedical science is driven by two equally pressing imperatives: a disinterested pursuit of knowledge for the sake of knowledge and a disinterested goal to do no harm. While generally the two imperatives coincide, they can come in conflict with one another in cases where the benefits may be substantial but consent may not have been secured or where a covert method is required for the study goals.

Hence, the second *Tri-council Policy Statement*, which governs the ethical protocol for the major funding bodies in Canada, allows deception and partial disclosure only in instances where such methods are necessary for viable research findings – often in psychological studies – where the study process does not put participants at risk of harm, and only if the participants are informed of their participation in the study and are given the opportunity to provide informed consent prior to the end of the research.[20] Adriana Petryna argues that an emphasis on consent has reduced the issue of ethics in contemporary clinical research to a procedural matter of getting bureaucratic approval from a research ethics board and obtaining the signed document that guarantees consent. The result is that the notion of ethics is subject to variance across different bureaucratic spaces, such as a research institution, a business firm, and regulatory bodies of different nation-states, each with its own set of struggles and field effects from different economic and political spaces.[21]

Not only is ethics in biomedicine a question of adherence to a bureaucratic procedure, but it is also a moving target, subject to interpretation and a practical strategy within this field. In the case of the Plan B story, the *CMAJ* owners found themselves in an awkward position in relation to the Canadian Pharmaceutical Association. The CPhA was upset by Eggertson and Sibbald's implication that it had engaged in unethical prescription practices, an accusation that could seriously harm the profession's reputation. Thus, the journal owners tried to block the story by declaring that it was scientifically unethical, not objective, and unscientific. Yet they neglected to subject the surveys conducted by the Canadian Pharmacists Association to the same ethical standard, nor did they point out the ethics of collecting testimonials from the women in the original story without written consent. The journal owners' glossing over these questions of ethics is not so much an ethical oversight as it is part of the strategic practice of ethics. Laura Stark demonstrates through her analysis of ethics review boards that decisions regarding the ethical viability of research studies involving human subjects, especially those studies whose designs do not fall neatly into existing protocols and regulations, can vary depending on institutional memory, which is composed of prior decisions made by individual boards.[22] Despite efforts at standardization and consistency, ethics review boards rely on group consideration, or the evaluation of a study design prior to the study by a group of research colleagues. This process necessarily opens up the possibility for debate and negotiation of what is and what is not ethical, depending on one's disciplinary priorities and personal moral concerns. Decisions about research ethics can hinge on the successful rhetoric of particular ethics panel members. Hence, ethics is as much a strategy in a field of struggles as it is a question of fixed ideals.

In addition to ethics, objectivity was also subject to different understanding by the *CMAJ* editors and owners, based on how journalism and science measure and assess that concept. Jeremy Iggers notes that, in journalism, there are two types of objectivity: one that reflects a realist position that measures objectivity by a journalist's ability to represent a pre-existing reality as fact, and the other that is not necessarily based in a clear epistemological grounding but in which objectivity is measured by how well a journalist follows a set of accepted procedures.[23] Lorraine Daston and Peter Galison show that a tension has always existed in Western science between the realist notion of truth and an ongoing epistemological problem of how best to represent it.[24] Debates and innovations in science are marked by changes in procedural criteria for establishing scientific objectivity. In general, the two journalists and the editors of the *CMAJ* argued that their ethical obligation lay in their public responsibility to uncover the truth about the practices of the Canadian Pharmacists Association. The journal owners framed objectivity as a procedural matter and ethics as a scientific responsibility to follow the procedures dictated by the field of biomedicine. These differing standards of objectivity were further complicated by the different procedures for ensuring objectivity in journalism and science.

The Plan B incident drew the curtain away from a set of compromises and struggles between science and journalism in medical reporting. Journalism entertains hypotheses and untested ideas, while science requires much more extensive testing. Despite their opposing standards, the science and journalism coexist in medical publishing more or less harmoniously, except in instances like the Plan B story where their fundamental incompatibility is revealed. The journal owners claimed that the Plan B story had no place in the journal because it was illegitimate scientific research. They argued that the report itself was conducted as scientific research and, therefore, had to meet the standards of peer-reviewed ethical research on human subjects. The editors of the journal claimed that the Plan B story had a place in the journal because it was legitimate journalistic reporting. They argued that the report was not based on scientific research and therefore had to meet the standards of journalistic reporting, which the original story did. Both the owners and the editors grounded their respective arguments on notions of truthfulness and objectivity but drew on different standards: science and journalism.

The owners never went as far as to claim that news reports should be eliminated from the contents of the journal altogether, but in demanding that news meet the standards of scientific research, they questioned the professional values of journalism and their appropriateness for medical reporting. Similarly, the editors and their supporters never went so far as to argue that the rules of journalism should override those of medical research. The ad hoc JOC argued that, "although investigative reporting was not part of the original activities of the *CMAJ* (and does not figure prominently in the journal even now), ... it is consistent with the journal's founding aim of providing a fresh and hence potentially corrective view."[25] At the same time, the JOC made a very clear distinction between journalism and science:

> The report (both as it was intended to be published and as it eventually appeared) does not meet the definition of "research" as understood in medical science. It is not systematic, is not generalizable, and makes no pretense of statistical analysis. In no way does it fit into a "grey area." It self-evidently fits within the norms of news investigation, not of scientific research, and its presentation within the news section of the journal makes its identity unambiguous.[26]

The JOC claimed that investigative reporting aligned with the overall values of the *CMAJ* and that the Plan B report fit the norms of journalism, not biomedical research. Despite a fundamental difference between medical research and journalism, there still remained an impetus to position medical publishing unproblematically between these two worlds. Yet it is precisely the tension between them that spurred the debate surrounding the Plan B story.

The position of both the journal owners and the editors shows that they were in fact in agreement that objectivity as a moral and technical value is central to medical science and medical publishing. Where they disagreed was with respect to the specific strategies by which one upholds this value within science. For the journal owners, who occupied an administrative role in science, this meant ensuring that the rules of science remained superior to those of journalism, even if it meant violating editorial autonomy. For the journal editors and their supporters, upholding objectivity meant a responsibility to uncover truth, even if it meant allowing the rules of journalism, an inferior field, to enter into medicine. In their own ways, both the owners and editors took risks to exert their own interpretation of what it meant to exercise objectivity.

In Defence of Objectivity

The disagreement about the Plan B story was but one incident in the mounting tensions between the journal editors and owners. In 2001, Hoey had run an editorial that supported the use of medical marijuana,[27] contrary to the CMA's official position on the substance. Shortly before their dismissal, the editors ran an editorial that criticized the newly appointed federal minister of health, Tony Clement, for his support of privatized medicine,[28] much to the embarrassment of the CMA. In making these decisions, the editors sought to engage with what they saw as socially and politically pertinent issues for Canadian medicine, while the journal owners wanted to maintain what they perceived to be a socially and politically neutral position with regard to controversial issues. The two sides struggled to position themselves as the champion of medical disinterestedness and objectivity, while critiquing the other for working against these tenets. In the process, the two sides drew on rhetorical strategies and interpretations of medical disinterestedness from the profession's past – nineteenth-century rules for gentlemanly battles of words and mid-twentieth-century priorities around the social role of medicine – in order to secure their own vision of the meaning of objectivity and the role of medical publishing in general.

While most of the disagreements between the journal editors and owners over editorial content took place behind the doors through departmental memos and phone conversations, the disputes over a 2002 editorial took place on the pages of the *CMAJ*. The editors highlighted a high-profile case in which a man died of cardiac arrest in a Quebec emergency room, largely due to understaffing. The man's death spurred the passing of a provincial bill that placed physicians under more demanding schedules and rigorous surveillance.[29] The editors argued that this political move by the provincial government resulted in a breach of trust between physicians and the government, although they briefly noted that physicians were obligated to their patients by bonds of trust and that "physicians broke that trust by not staffing the ED of such an important regional hospital," a failure that resulted in the death of a patient.[30] The CMA's president at the time, Dana Hanson, argued that the editorial's claim that "physicians have betrayed the trust" was unsubstantiated and "amounts to an unwarranted attack on the whole profession." He concluded that the editorial was "seriously flawed" and "repugnant" and that "our colleagues in Quebec deserve a retraction."[31] The entire editorial board responded to Hanson's letter under the banner of editorial independence, calling it a sign of "clear and present danger" for "the right to articulate such opinions without concern for retribution by an organization or corporation that holds ownership or operating responsibility for the journal."[32] In the next issue of the journal, Hanson withdrew his demand for the retraction of the editorial.

The conflict between the CMA president and the editorial board harkens back to editorial sparring in nineteenth-century medical journals, where the two sides of the duel of words claimed a disinterested position by demonstrating flaws in the other's claim to medical disinterestedness. At stake in these exchanges was the author's honour as a gentleman and, later, the honour of the profession. While the 2002 version of the duel of words in the *CMAJ* lacked the gender and class inflections of the nineteenth-century discourse of gentlemanliness, the rhetoric followed a similar structure and style. Each side sought to portray themselves as calm, cool, and collected while positioning the other as irrational, unreasonable, and going against the interests of the profession at large.

At stake in the dispute between the editorial board and the CMA president was objectivity: by accusing the other of going against objectivity, each side tried to position itself as morally and scientifically superior. Hanson sought to avoid political conflict among the constituents of his professional body by taking the position of standing up for his colleagues from undue criticism, while also denouncing the actions of the editorial board as dishonourable. Both the Quebec editorial and the Plan B story placed the CMA in uncomfortable situations where it had to deal with retaliations from powerful professional and political groups such as the Quebec Medical Association, the federal government, and the Canadian Pharmacists Association. The journal owners strove to portray the editors as biased in order to more generally claim that opinions about controversial issues did not have a rightful place in medical publishing. For example, in his letter, the CMA president used words such as "betrayed the trust," "unwarranted attack," and "repugnant" in order to brand the opinion of the editors as extreme, unsubstantiated, and base – and not objective. In response to Hanson's attack, the editorial board accused him of attempting to violate editorial autonomy. By calling out the CMA president's act of transgression against professional interests in maintaining objectivity, the editors positioned themselves as defenders of objectivity.

The editorial board's accusation fell on sympathetic ears. When the management of the *CMAJ* was privatized, there were concerns that external pressures, such as the pharmaceutical industry and other major advertisers in the journal, could compromise the journal's contents.[33] A March 2006 editorial stated that the "integrity of the knowledge is being corroded by commercial interests" in Canadian medicine,[34] alerting readers to the perceived threat of market forces to the science of medicine. The firings at the *JAMA* and the *NEJM* also placed the *CMAJ* editors on high alert. Supporters of the *CMAJ* editors often turned to historicized narratives that medical journals have always had "an important watchdog function by challenging the forces that undermine the values of medicine."[35] Hanson was compelled to retract his position because the disagreement took place during a time in medical publishing when editorial autonomy was already a heated issue and a site where objectivity had to be defended.

The CMA president's position was positioned as threatening to the ideal of objectivity.

The journal owners and editors adopted positions that were in keeping with interpretations of medical disinterestedness at different moments in the history of professional medicine in Canada. Owners insisted on maintaining harmonious relations with other groups, in keeping with the CMA president's goal in 1963 to build bridges with the public, governments, and the media[36] – worlds outside of the intellectual field of medicine – as a way to effectively convey the disinterested intentions of doctors. The owners mobilized the professional ethic of public relations by avoiding controversial social issues and overt criticisms about other professional associations and the government in power. Meanwhile, the editors drew on the nineteenth century's legacy of medical journals as forums for disputes between medical men over questions of what constituted a learned profession (which included socially charged issues such as French-British relations). The editors and their supporters especially deferred to Thomas Wakley, the controversial founder of the *Lancet*, who highlighted malpractice (at a time when medical men were trying to forge a brotherhood) and disseminated scientific knowledge to less privileged rural medical men, much to the dismay of his more conservative peers in the cities.[37] The *CMAJ* editors and their supporters drew on the position of medical men of the nineteenth century who upheld the democratic ideals of science in order to instigate medical and social reform.

Both sides of the dispute mobilized different articulations of medical disinterestedness that had been acceptable at various times in the history of the profession. The long-term disputes between the *CMAJ* editors and owners show that different statements of and claims to medical disinterestedness gain traction and credibility according to the historical context in which they are made. For instance, while effective public relations was characterized as a morally justifiable move in the aftermath of the Saskatchewan doctors' strike in the 1960s, the twenty-first-century medical community judged the *CMAJ* owners' use of public relation strategies to lack objectivity and violate editorial autonomy. In addition to being historically specific, collective judgments about what doctors ought and ought not to do contain within them moral tensions and pitfalls. While the journal owners insisted that controversial social and political issues did not have a legitimate place in medical publishing, the early *Lancet* contained very little science and was, in fact, a vehicle to raise controversy and to entertain physicians and the public (the early *British Medical Journal (BMJ)* was also more interested in promoting the profession than in disseminating scientific research).[38] Indeed, nineteenth-century Canadian medical journals were forums for heated socio-political battles between medical men, and the *CMAJ* of the 1950s and 1960s contained editorials and essays on medical reform that often delved into competing political philosophies.

Meanwhile, editorial autonomy, which the journal editors upheld as sacred to the intellectual and democratic values of science, was not a fail-safe concept. Richard Smith, a former editor-in-chief of the *BMJ*, cautions that editorial decisions often receive little monitoring and that "little progress had been made in a decade to develop ways to respond to editorial misconduct."[39] He argues that, while journal owners have the legal right to interfere in cases of editorial misconduct, there is no clear-cut line between misconduct and legitimate conduct. In fact, he claims that "editors are expected to discriminate, but they should discriminate on grounds of evidence, importance, relevance, quality and clarity rather than on personal foibles. But it is also widely believed to be the job of the editor to give a publication a 'personality' – and that's likely to be related to his or her personality. So some personal selection seems desirable."[40]

The notion of "personality," which Smith places in air quotes, contrasts with the subject- and personality-free notions of "evidence, importance, relevance, quality and clarity," demonstrating that there is a tension between the standards of objectivity and the expectations of creativity in editorialship. Smith's description of editors suggests that medical publishing is messy and amorphous and cannot be guided by an inherent objectivity according to scientific or journalistic rules, or by the subjectivity of the editor alone. Instead, the overall trustworthiness of a medical journal is made possible by the figure of the editor, who embodies the scientific dispositions of the medical habitus, but who can still exercise creativity and innovation within the range of what is possible and thinkable in medical publishing. Smith's stance on the scientific and disinterested role of the editor is also reflected in his conclusion that "we have no good data, only stories, but I suspect that cases of editors performing poorly far outnumber cases of frank misconduct,"[41] a statement that highlights not only the difficulty in distinguishing explicit and intentional (mis)conduct from unintentional and well-intended (mis)conduct, but also the inherent ambiguity and flexibility in the criteria for scientific objectivity.

The owners and the editors of the *CMAJ* both struggled to defend and maintain their own version of objectivity as the dominant norm in the journal. The editors drew on the value of editorial autonomy, while the owners advocated that engaging in direct social and political debates was not the proper realm of medical publishing. The rhetorical strategies of both sides took on a highly moralized tinge, suggesting that questions of good science are embedded in a social struggle over the power to define what objectivity means (and what it does not mean). This struggle is fought and won by effectively mobilizing already acceptable discourses of medical disinterestedness, and the historical context in which claims to objectivity are made can arbitrate which claims are deemed truly disinterested. Out of this struggle, or conflicting interests in what objectivity should mean, emerges articulations of what objectivity means and does not mean – definitions that can be revised or upturned in another struggle over conflicting ideas of medical disinterestedness.

Separation of Science and Business
The result of the disputes between the *CMAJ* editors and owners reverberated across Canadian medicine. Sixteen of eighteen other members of the *CMAJ* editorial board resigned to express solidarity with John Hoey. The interim senior editor, Stephen Choi, resigned from the position one week after his appointment.[42] While the subsequent interim editor of the journal, Noni MacDonald, claimed that the controversies were blown out of proportion,[43] negative publicity against the CMA mounted. The Canadian media, including the *Globe and Mail* and the Canadian Broadcasting Corporation, consistently reported on the events in a way that criticized the CMA. Potential contributors to the journal withheld their submissions, claiming that they were unable to trust the journal's integrity – "I feel no compelling reason to do *pro bono* research for a CMA mouthpiece," said one writer[44] – or that they would rather

submit their article to a more stable journal.[45] There was a very real fear that the reputation of the journal was on the line, which would greatly threaten the legitimacy of the CMA itself and the reputation of Canadian medicine in general.

The incident made uncomfortably, and even dangerously, explicit what had been an implicit and unspoken reality of medical publishing – that the business of publishing coexists with the intellectual work of science. After the dismissal, the owners of the *CMAJ* and the dismissed editors came up with different solutions to the problem of the tainted image of Canadian medical publishing. The CMA established an external review panel to investigate the governance of the *CMAJ*, in an attempt to salvage the journal's reputation from the wreckage of the high-profile controversy. The dismissed editors founded a new open-source medical journal as a way to set their own terms of editorialship. Both moves represented strategies that reflected their advocates' respective positions on how best to protect and enact objectivity in medical publishing. Yet both relied on relatively vague criteria of trust and good faith in the editorial and ownership structures as a way to ensure that the business of medical publishing remained separate from the intellectual work of science.

The CMA appointed a Governance Review Panel, which in July 2006 made a set of recommendations: (1) to return the ownership of the journal to the CMA board of directors and not under the management of CMA Holdings, which was a private corporation; (2) to make explicit the role and composition of the Journal Oversight Committee, with each member serving for a fixed term (a maximum of three years), with members being drawn from the CMA board from a shortlist of candidates provided by the existing JOC, and with a freelance journalist being included on the committee; (3) to mandate that the JOC respond within forty-eight to seventy-two hours of a complaint and be granted the full authority to arbitrate in cases of editorial conflict; (4) to cap the maximum term of the editor-in-chief at five years (Hoey served ten years before he was dismissed); and (5) to divide the duties of the editor-in-chief into two separate streams – management of journal content through the JOC and of journal business through the CMA board, in order to ensure editorial independence and organizational transparency.[46] The panel's recommendations, which the CMA adopted, generally envisioned an organizational restructuring of the conditions of journal ownership and editorialship and of the relationship between the two streams. What was clearly absent in the panel's report were explicit rules to "'publish this, but not that.'"[47] Instead, the report stressed that the owners and editors had to be able "to work together in a spirit of mutual trust and collaboration," while claiming that "trust and good faith cannot be mandated" or written as rules.[48] The implication was that it was impossible to impose explicit rules to govern the relationship between the editorial board and the CMA. Indeed, rules were not truly desirable because they would be antithetical to the democratic ideals of scientific work and the disinterested ideal of scientific knowledge as a natural and cumulative progression. Rules might also introduce forces that were external to the logic of the scientific field, such as political pressures and conflicts.

Yet, restructuring the conditions under which the intellectual work of scientific medicine could be conducted in a disinterested manner was not entirely derived from a purely intellectual goal to ensure objectivity and neutrality. It was a strategic move to salvage Canadian medical publishing from a crisis of faith among those who were invested in the journal as an objective enterprise – contributors, researchers, reviewers, readers, and the public. Amir Attaran, a professor of law and population health who served on the Governance Review Panel, claimed that "these and other recommendations by the panel will help to avoid the ultimate criticism: that the *CMAJ* is only a house organ for the CMA."[49] His specific reference to the need to avoid criticism, rather than to proactively ensure objectivity and neutrality, is evocative of Gaye Tuchman's study of journalistic objectivity as a ritualized strategy – "tactics used offensively to anticipate attack or defensively [to] deflect criticism"[50] – in the struggle to claim truthfulness. The dismissal of the *CMAJ* editors placed the administrative aspects of the intellectual work of medical science under the spotlight, resulting in an uncomfortable and problematic situation for Canadian medical publishing, in which its scientificness and medical disinterestedness were put into question. To remedy the situation, the best that the panel could do was to cordon off intellectual science from the business of medical journals, symbolized by its recommendation to include a more prominent disclaimer that the editorial contents did not necessarily reflect the CMA's views and policies.[51] Neither the panel nor the CMA went as far as to completely eliminate the business aspects of the journal, nor did they claim to do so. However, by increasing the distance between the intellectual work of science (encapsulated by editorial independence) and the administrative work of the scientific institution (represented by the CMA board that oversaw the business side of publishing) as much as possible, the journal owners could claim that editorial autonomy remained unhindered by economic and political forces, thereby restoring the journal's reputation and the CMA's own international professional standing as an objective group.

The business side of medical publishing returned to being an acceptable compromise and a necessary evil in the production of scientific medicine: the implicit but unspoken reality was that business and science coexisted in medical publishing. The journal rendered the incident as a temporary problem that was quickly resolved: "Already, *CMAJ*'s new governance structure is being recognized by other associations as a model for journal publishing, a strong signal of the importance and visionary nature of the Governance Review Panel's work."[52] What had been a controversy that shook the very foundations of intellectual medicine in Canada became absorbed into the continuity of medical history and progress. The review panel had deemed that a mere structural separation of the administrative side and the intellectual work of medical publishing was sufficient to legitimately present medical research in a disinterested and objective manner.

While the CMA struggled to improve the organizational structure of the *CMAJ*, Hoey, Todkill, and their colleagues abandoned the idea of the salvageability of the *CMAJ* and founded *Open Medicine* under a Creative Commons licence.[53] Editorial independence and the ownership of medical knowledge became the primary lenses through which the editors framed their rationale for founding *Open Medicine*. They emphasized that "medical knowledge should be public and free from undeclared influence" and that the contents of the journal "will be 'owned' by all who read and contribute to it."[54] These rhetorical and organizational moves were based on debates within the *CMAJ* and among international medical journals that had developed over the years. The editors believed that medical associations do not own journals but are custodians of them and cannot interfere with intellectual work: "Any medical journal belongs, intellectually and morally, to its contributors, editors, editorial boards and readers – a sort of constituent assembly. It also belongs to the world: the dissemination of medical science is, or should be, ultimately a humanitarian project, and not merely the special preserve of professional associations."[55] This vision drew on the Enlightenment ideals of scientificness – progress, humanism, communalism, and equality. Those ideals had underpinned the Victorian scientificness that had greatly influenced Canadian medical men's struggle to regulate membership into the profession. More than a century later, these ideals were reimagined to outline the conditions under which knowledge production and dissemination may be deemed scientific.

While the CMA sought to regain the faith of the *CMAJ*'s readership and contributors by structurally distancing the business from the intellectual work of science, the editors of *Open Medicine* did away altogether with the business aspects of publishing that run so contrary to the disinterested logic of intellectual science. Their position was that the "noneconomic benefits" would offset any financial losses (arising from a lack of revenue from print subscriptions and advertising) by allowing a "wider dissemination of scholarly and scientific content,"[56] the ultimate goal of a truly disinterested intellectual enterprise. The disinterested logic was extended to instances of editorial misconduct, which was to be assessed as a violation of intellectual standards, rather than as a political or financial transgression, so that the misconduct could be assessed within the scientific community of editors, writers, and readers.

However, there are problems deep within the editorial process that have little to do with journal ownership. Richard Smith points to the serious gap in knowledge and training when editors first come on board, which results in inconsistencies: "most editors of the world's 10,000 or so biomedical journals have received no training," and "many editors work largely alone" even though "editing ... is becoming steadily more complex."[57] While some editorial training was available, particularly through the World Association of Medical Editors, it was extremely limited, and "most editors still learn on the job."[58] The Committee on Publication Ethics and the International Medical Scientific Press Council were established to monitor editorial accountability, but both are organized to respond to complaints and have significant procedural problems;

moreover, no disciplinary measures are in place other than removal from the organizations themselves.[59] The editorial policies of *Open Medicine* did not directly address these issues, nor did they lay out rigid rules of conduct. Instead, they relied on the skills, commitment, and good faith of a volunteer-based board who pledged to "support the Editor-in-Chief(s) to maintain Journal principles underlying the editorial integrity and independence of the Journal" – namely, "editorial independence, Journal advertising policies and the open access platform."[60] The accountability of the editor-in-chief was to be ensured by an annual meeting to "review a report on the performance of the Editor-in-Chief from the Chair of the Board of Directors."[61] The position of *Open Medicine* demonstrates an appeal to the rationalism of the group and an emphasis on trust and good faith in the individual members of the board in order to establish and maintain the scientificness and medical disinterestedness of the journal's editorialship.

According to Daston and Galison, a community of scientific individuals forms symbolic relations based on "trained judgment," which is the form that objectivity has taken in the twentieth century.[62] In the nineteenth century, it became impossible to defer to an external reality unhindered by human subjectivity as a way to claim an objective scientific observation. In the twentieth century, the notion of a scientific subjectivity that was inclined to suppress itself through proper training allowed Western science to bypass the problem of the subjectivity of the observer. In other words, a fully inculcated scientific habitus resolved the issue of maintaining a standard of objectivity across scientific practices. Similarly, the terms of reference of *Open Medicine* relied on an honour system in which the scientific aptitude of an individual editor could be ensured through the structural processes of medical education, research, and board selection, with trust and good faith, not explicit and rigid rules of conduct, governing the editorial board.

Thus, the two opposing sides of the controversy, the journal owners and the dismissed editors, both relied on a loosely defined honour code to rectify what was perceived as a broken system and to emerge from the highly publicized crisis with their scientific reputation intact. While the two groups disagreed about the role and mandate of the medical journal, to the point of severing ties, they in fact equally relied on modifying organizational processes to mend and restructure relationships between the editors-in-chief, the editorial board, the board of directors, and the readership, rather than erecting a code of rules that explicitly outlined what could and could not be done. The separation of the administrative aspects of science and the intellectual work of science opened up different positions from which to claim objectivity and scientific disinterestedness. In the case of the *CMAJ*, creating a structural divide between the editorial board and the business of a journal, and being very public about this bureaucratic separation, could mend the journal's reputation enough to attract submissions and readers once more. For *Open Medicine*, by completely abandoning a profit-based business model and opening the journal management to a group of like-minded physicians, this group of editors could uphold editorial autonomy as evidence of the journal's objectivity, while holding at bay the fundamental fragility of editorialship.

In both instances, scientific disinterestedness operated as procedural objectivity – a defensive mechanism to deflect criticism and to keep misconduct at bay. Both solutions relied on a social understanding among the players, or "good faith" between professionals, with the bureaucratic structures providing some framework around which to act with decorum and with disinterest. Neither solution would prove to be lasting, however. In 2016, another editor-in-chief was fired from the *CMAJ* under mysterious circumstances, reopening concerns about editorial autonomy, objectivity, and the feasibility of medical publishing in general.[63] In 2014, *Open Medicine* folded, citing persistent funding issues and the challenges of relying on a volunteer editorial board.[64] There have been new threats as well, including recent scandals around two publishers of Canadian medical journals being bought by a company reputed to publish "junk science."[65] With these existing and new challenges, the tension between the disinterested pursuit of "pure" medical science and the economic realities of communicating this knowledge remains ever present.

***

The dismissal of the senior editors of the *CMAJ* in 2006 and the events surrounding it demonstrate that its significance went beyond the violation of editorial autonomy. In embracing media work, medicine took advantage of the publishing infrastructure of media industries, but, in doing so, medicine opened itself up to the forces of media and journalism, including fundamentally different, though not necessarily incompatible, standards of ethics and objectivity. Indeed, in the conflicts surrounding the Plan B story, we see how it was possible for the journal editors to make ethical claims that were acceptable in journalism but not in medicine, yet still garner support. The two sides of the struggle – the journal editors and owners – also drew on various claims from different time periods about what medicine ought to be in order to support their interests in what ought to be (and ought not to be) covered in the *CMAJ*. The struggle also raised questions about what medical professionals' role ought to be in relation to political and social issues – that is, whether to take a position and advocate for others or remain neutral. These questions were framed as defining issues related to medical disinterestedness, all the while inflected by each side's stake in controlling the direction of the journal.

Ultimately, objectivity and ethics could be shaped and argued in accordance with the interests of those who claimed to be objective and ethical in the name of medical disinterestedness, with differing levels of success. The journal owners fired editors who were a thorn in their side by calling the editors' actions unethical, but then faced accusations of violating editorial autonomy. The journal editors were fired but won the support of the international medical community. Both the owners and editors came up with solutions to salvage and protect objectivity and ethics in Canadian medical publishing, by creating separate business and editorial streams and by founding a fully open source journal, respectively. Neither strategy did away with the fundamental issue of having to rely on media and economic forces to publish medical knowledge. Then, as now, medical knowledge production remains open to forces outside of science proper, including ethical norms of other fields, such as journalism, and economic forces of media industries.

Conclusion

Moral, ethical, and scientific standards in medicine have often emerged and taken shape in direct relation to issues of conflict of interest. Questions of what doctors ought and ought not do in the name of medical disinterestedness have been posed and answered in the midst of struggles for professional medicine to secure and maintain its authority and legitimacy as experts in all matters of health and illness vis-à-vis other groups – the state, the media, and the general public – invested in how medicine is done. Particularly in moments where these other groups called into question the moral or scientific credibility of medicine, doctors articulated their claims to disinterestedness in ways that shaped what it means to be medical professionals acting on behalf of patients, the public, and the pursuit of scientific knowledge.

In the nineteenth century, doctors in Canada formed their professional identity around what it legitimately meant to be a doctor of high moral and scientific standing. The medical professional identity coalesced around the idealized figure of the British physician gentleman, which was mobilized to delegitimate other health professions, such as Thompsonians, and restrict the entry of "undesirables," such as French Canadians and graduates from American and Canadian medical schools, into the profession. The newly emerging medical profession strove to align its professional interests, such as autonomy and dominance over other health professions, with the public's interest in receiving the best remedies from trustworthy healers who had the patient's best interest at heart. The figure of the gentleman physician sat at the juncture of these two interests by guaranteeing respectability and trustworthiness via the moral pedigree of his social class and the scientific credibility of his education.

In the mid-twentieth century, the joining of professional and public interest under the rubric of medical disinterestedness unravelled when the medical profession in Saskatchewan contested the provincial government's proposal for a tax-funded, government-administered health insurance program. The profession and the government posited differing conceptualization of health – a private contract between a physician and a patient versus the right of all citizens – and each argued that they were the most appropriate body to ensure its appropriate administration and protection. When the profession faced criticism from the national press for opposing a health care plan based on social welfare, it scrambled to regain public trust as a moral profession, claiming that it had always acted in the interest of the public but had miscommunicated its disinterested intentions. By way of a solution, the profession strengthened family practice and its representation in public health, two fading disciplines in medicine at the time, as the more humane face of medicine while establishing a presence in the media and public relations to reflect and promote its socially responsibility.

The final historical case discussed in this book was the controversial sacking in 2006 of the editors-in-chief at the top-ranking medical journal in Canada. The incident and the surrounding discourse showed that standards of objectivity and ethics in medical publishing are constantly negotiated and debated at the troubling intersection between the intellectual science of medicine and the business of publishing. This tension is fundamental to the production and dissemination of medical knowledge – even in open-source publishing, which faces different financing challenges. To respond to international accusations that editorial autonomy at the journal had been transgressed and to remedy the crisis of faith in the integrity of Canadian medical publishing, the journal board and owners created a bureaucratic barrier between the work of medical science proper and business administration, a temporary solution that has invited, and will likely continue to invite, future conflicts between the scientific interests and business priorities of the journal.

The three historical cases show how the solutions proposed to resolve a moral or scientific controversy in medicine laid the groundwork for new ethical and scientific problems. Nineteenth-century doctors raised their moral profile in relation to other health practitioners by claiming that they were acting in a disinterested manner on behalf of public health, although they still expected to be paid for services rendered. The issue of payment became the subject of heated conflict between the medical profession and the government of Saskatchewan in the context of the latter's proposal for health reform, resulting in the profession being shamed in the media for acting selfishly without regard for public welfare. The profession embraced media and public relations as a way to mend its damaged reputation and relationship with the public, but opening the door to the media industry also opened medicine up to the forces of media and their industries. In medical publishing, industry pressures of financing and circulation butted up against the imperative to disseminate objective and ethical content.

These cases show how invested disinterestedness – or the moral claim and conviction to act on behalf of something or someone other than the self – is never neat or complete. It cannot be. Invested disinterestedness is fundamentally about contradictions and tensions. In medicine, there is an incompatibility between doctors' claims (and collective belief) to have in their hearts the interests of the public and patients, over and above their own interests, and doctors' desire and need to be paid for their services, dictate the conditions of their work, have authority over matters of health and illness, and rely on business forces to publish and disseminate medical knowledge. The two interests coexist but are at odds with one another, although most of the time doctors tolerate the tension as a necessary evil or a manageable conflict of interest. In certain moments, however, as in the historical examples examined in this book, the contradiction between the two interests is so severe that doctors as a group cannot but confront the double truth about their claim to invested disinterestedness – that they (expect to) benefit from their actions that they claim are on behalf of something greater than themselves.

Yet, even in these moments when the double truth of invested disinterestedness could not be ignored, the entire institution and culture of medicine did not collapse under the weight of its own contradictions. Despite the internal contradictions of acting on behalf of something and someone other than the self, doctors as a group collectively believe that the work of medicine as a moral and scientific enterprise is worthwhile – or, to put it in Bourdieu's terms, that the game is worth playing. The medical habitus is robust enough to weather the contradictions inherent in invested disinterestedness and to maintain the collective belief that objective and ethical medical practice is possible and necessary, even if these ideals are constantly under threat by forces that are less than objective or ethical. This belief has compelled the medical profession to repeatedly rearticulate what it means to be invested in disinterestedness, and to restructure its institutions and structures accordingly when confronted with accusations that doctors are not as morally or scientifically upright as they claim.

We all have a stake in having medicine aspire to be as objective and ethical as possible – we are all patients at some point in our lives, and we all want the best care possible, based on the most objective scientific knowledge, provided by medical practitioners with the best moral intentions.[1] To hold institutions that insist on their disinterestedness accountable to their claims, we must understand how doctors, like many others who navigate complex moral questions, are able to suspend their moral judgment and how they can give the benefit of the doubt to those who make morally questionable choices or dismiss a moral transgression as reflecting the lesser of two evils or as a case of the ends justifying the means. We can ask what kinds of discursive moves and what kinds of distancing strategies at the bureaucratic level of organizations allow medical professionals to inhabit morally ambiguous positions more or less comfortably. As is evident in the three historical cases examined in this book, high-profile instances of moral or scientific transgressions are often the tip of the iceberg – spectacular manifestations of more deeply seated, long-standing, and everyday moral and scientific tensions that go unnoticed and are often made possible by other moral and scientific compromises and acquiescence from previous times. Rather than merely determine the presence or absence of conflict of interest, we can also focus on how different, and at times conflicting, ideas of medical disinterestedness are articulated, discussed, and navigated. We can also ask what other interests and forces are ignored or accepted without question. It is in the messy and uncomfortable spaces where the line between "ought" and "ought not" are blurred that medicine's moral and scientific standards are made and remade.

Notes

Introduction

1 See Michael Oldani, "Thick Prescriptions: Toward an Interpretation of Pharmaceutical Sales Practices," *Medical Anthropology Quarterly* 18, 3 (2004): 324–56; Joel Lexchin, "Those Who Have the Gold Make the Evidence: How the Pharmaceutical Industry Biases the Outcomes of Clinical Trials of Medications," *Science and Engineering Ethics* 18, 2 (2012): 247–61; Sergio Sismondo, "Ghosts in the Machine: Publication Planning in the Medical Sciences," *Social Studies of Science* 39, 2 (2009): 171–98; K.J. Holloway, "Teaching Conflict: Professionalism and Medical Education," *Journal of Bioethical Inquiry* 12, 4 (2015): 675–85.

2 S.E.D. Shortt presents an excellent review of this early literature in "Antiquarians and Amateurs: Reflections on the Writing of Medical History in Canada" in his *Medicine in Canadian Society: Historical Perspectives* (Montreal/Kingston: McGill-Queen's University Press, 1981), 1–18.

3 Canniff begins his text with "the conquest of General Wolfe in 1759" and the American War of Independence. He emphasizes that "as with the other learned professions, the cream of the medical men in the several revolting colonies remained loyal to the British flag." William Canniff, *The Medical Profession in Upper Canada, 1783–1850: An Historical Narrative with Original Documents relating to the Profession including Some Brief Biographies* (Toronto: William Briggs, 1894), 12.

4 R.D. Gidney and W.P.J. Millar, "The Origins of Organized Medicine in Ontario, 1850–1869," in *Health, Disease and Medicine: Essays in Canadian History*, ed. C.G. Roland, 65–95 (Toronto: Hannah Institute for the History of Medicine, 1984); Barbara R. Tunis, "Medical Licensing in Lower Canada: The Disputes over Canada's First Medical Degree," in Shortt, *Medicine in Canadian Society*, 137–64; Hilda

Neatby, "The Medical Profession in the North-West Territories," in Shortt, *Medicine in Canadian Society*, 165–88; Veronica Strong-Boag, "Canada's Women Doctors: Feminism Constrained," in Shortt, *Medicine in Canadian Society*, 207–36; Barbara Tunis, "Medical Education and Medical Licensing in Lower Canada: Demographic Factors, Conflict and Social Change," *Histoire sociale/Social History* 27 (May 1981): 67–91; Sylvio Leblond, "La médecine dans la province de Québec avant 1847," *Les cahier des dix* 35 (1970): 65–95.

5 Colin D. Howell, "Elite Doctors and the Development of Scientific Medicine: The Halifax Medical Establishment and 19th Century Medical Professionalism," in Roland, *Health, Disease and Medicine*, 106–8.

6 S.E.D. Shortt, "'Before the Age of Miracles': The Rise, Fall and Rebirth of General Practice in Canada, 1890–1940," in Roland, *Health, Disease and Medicine*, 123–52; Howell, "Elite Doctors," 105–22; Geoffrey Bilson, "Canadian Doctors and the Cholera," in Shortt, *Medicine in Canadian Society*, 115–36.

7 S.E.D. Shortt, "Physicians, Science, and Status: Issues in the Professionalization of Anglo-American Medicine in the Nineteenth Century," *Medical History* 27 (1983): 52.

8 Ibid., 61.

9 Paul Underhill, "Alternative Views of Science in Intra-professional Conflict: General Practitioners and the Medical and Surgical Elite 1815–58," *Journal of Historical Sociology* 5, 3 (1992): 322–50.

10 Jaclyn Duffin, *History of Medicine: A Scandalously Short Introduction*, 2nd ed. (Toronto: University of Toronto Press, 2010).

11 Evan Willis, "Introduction: Taking Stock of Medical Dominance," *Health Sociology Review* 15 (2006): 421.

12 See David Coburn, George M. Torrance, and Joseph M. Kaufert, "Medical Dominance in Canada in Historical Perspective: The Rise and Fall of Medicine?" *International Journal of Health Services* 13, 3 (1983): 407–32; David Coburn, "Canadian Medicine: Dominance or Proletarianization?" *Milbank Quarterly* 66, Suppl. 2 (1988): 92–116; Deborah A. Stone, "The Doctor as Businessman: The Changing Politics of a Cultural Icon," *Journal of Health Politics, Policy and Law* 22, 2 (1997): 533–56; David Coburn, "State Authority, Medical Dominance, and Trends in the Regulation of Health Professions: The Ontario Case," *Social Science and Medicine* 37, 2 (1993): 129–38; Nicky Britten, "Prescribing and the Defense of Clinical Autonomy," *Sociology of Health and Illness* 23, 4 (2001): 478–96; John McKinlay and Joan Arches, "Towards the Proletarianization of Physicians," *International Journal of Health Services* 15 (1985): 161–95; Vicente Navarro, "Professional Dominance or Proletarianization? Neither," *Milbank Quarterly* 66, Suppl. 2 (1988): 57–75.

13 In this literature, the emphasis is on bodies and concepts that are medicalized, such as women's bodies, race, poverty, criminality, and so on; doctors may be agents of medicalization, particularly in doctor-patient interactions, in which they generally exercise authoritative power.

14 Ronald Hamowy, *Canadian Medicine: A Study in Restricted Entry* (Vancouver: Fraser Institute, 1984), 8.

15 Howard S. Becker et al., *Boys in White: Student Culture in Medical School* (New Brunswick, NJ: Transaction, 1977).

16 Haida Luke, *Medical Education and Sociology of Medical Habitus: "It's Not about the Stethoscope!"* (Boston: Kluwer Academic, 2003).

17 Renady Hightower, "Ethnography of the Habitus of the Emergency Physician" (PhD diss., Wayne State University, 2010).

18 See Becker et al., *Boys in White,* but also doctor-patient interaction studies such as Candace West, "When the Doctor Is a 'Lady': Power, Status and Gender in Physician-Patient Encounters," *Symbolic Interaction* 7, 1 (1984): 87–106, and Sally E. Thorne et al., "The Context of Health Care Communication in Chronic Illness," *Patient Education and Counseling* 54 (2004): 299–306.

19 Luke, *Medical Education.*

20 Ibid.

21 Sarah Nettleton, Roger Burrows, and Ian Watt, "Regulating Medical Bodies? The Consequences of the 'Modernisation' of the NHS and the Disembodiment of Clinical Knowledge," *Sociology of Health and Illness* 30, 3 (2008): 333–48.

22 David Armstrong and Jane Ogden, "The Role of Etiquette and Experimentation in Explaining How Doctors Change Behavior: A Qualitative Study," *Sociology of Health and Illness* 28, 7 (2006): 951–68.

23 David Armstrong, "Embodiment and Ethics: Constructing Medicine's Two Bodies," *Sociology of Health and Illness* 28, 6 (2006): 866–81.

24 Michel Foucault, *Madness and Civilization: A History of Insanity in the Age of Reason,* trans. Richard Howard (New York: Vintage Books, 1965); Michel Foucault, *The Birth of the Clinic: An Archaeology of Medical Perception,* trans. A.M. Sheridan (London: Routledge, 2003).

25 Thomas Osborne, "Medicine and Epistemology: Michel Foucault and the Liberality of Clinical Reason," *History of the Human Sciences* 5, 2 (1992): 63–93.

26 See Ian Hacking, *The Social Construction of What?* (Cambridge, MA: Harvard University Press: 1999); Annmarie Mol, *The Logic of Care: Health and the Problem of Patient Choice* (Abingdon, UK/New York: Routledge: 2008).

27 Lisa Cartwright, *Screening the Body: Tracing Medicine's Visual Culture* (Minneapolis: University of Minnesota Press, 1995); Paula Treichler, Lisa Cartwright, and Constance Penley, *The Visible Woman: Imaging Technologies, Gender, and Science* (New York: New York University Press, 1998); Anne Balsamo, *Technologies of the Gendered Body: Reading Cyborg Women* (Durham, NC: Duke University Press, 1996).

28 P. Lealle Ruhl, "Liberal Governance and Prenatal Care," *Economy and Society* 28 (1999): 95–117; Lorna Weir, *Pregnancy, Risk and Biopolitics: On the Threshold of the Living Subject* (London: Routledge, 2006); Suzanne Fraser and kylie valentine, *Substance and Substitution: Methadone Subjects in Liberal Societies* (New York/Basingstoke, UK: Palgrave Macmillan, 2008).

29 Nikolas Rose, *The Politics of Life Itself: Biomedicine, Power, and Subjectivity in the Twenty-First Century* (Princeton, NJ: Princeton University Press, 2007); Adriana Petryna, Andrew Lakoff, and Arthur Kleinman, eds., *Global Pharmaceuticals* (Durham, NC: Duke University Press, 2006); Samantha King, *Pink Ribbon, Inc.: Breast Cancer and the Politics of Philanthropy* (Minneapolis: University of Minnesota Press, 2006).

30 Cindy Patton, *Rebirth of the Clinic* (Minneapolis: University of Minnesota Press, 2010); Troy Duster, *Backdoor to Eugenics* (New York: Routledge, 2003); Bruno Latour, *Pasteurization of France*, trans. A. Sheridan and J. Law (Cambridge, MA: Harvard University Press, 1988).

31 Evelyn Hammonds, "Towards a Geneology of Black Female Sexuality: The Problematic Silence," in *Feminist Theory and the Body: A Reader*, ed. Janet Price and Margaret Shildrick, 245–59 (New York: Routledge, 1997); Adele Clarke and Virginia Olsen, *Revisioning Women, Health and Healing: Feminist, Cultural and Technoscience Perspectives* (New York: Routledge, 1999); Susan Wendell, *Rejected Body: Feminist Philosophical Reflections on Disability* (New York: Routledge, 1996).

32 Marc Berg and Annmarie Mol, eds., *Differences in Medicine: Unravelling Practices, Techniques and Bodies* (Durham, NC: Duke University Press, 1998); Cindy Patton and John Liesch, "In Your Face," in *Cosmetic Surgery: A Feminist Primer*, ed. Cressida J. Hayes and Meredith Jones, 209–24 (Farnham, UK/Burlington, VT: Ashgate, 2009); Sander L. Gilman, "AIDS and Syphilis: The Iconography of Disease," in *AIDS: Cultural Analysis/Cultural Activism*, ed. Douglas Crimp, 87–107 (Cambridge, MA: October Books, 1988); Jan Zita Grover, "AIDS: Keywords," in Crimp, *AIDS*, 17–30; Susan Sontag, *AIDS and Its Metaphors* (New York: Farrar, Straus and Giroux, 1989); Cindy Patton, *Sex and Germs: The Politics of AIDS* (Boston: South End Press, 1985); Cindy Patton, *Inventing AIDS* (New York: Routlege, 1990); Paula Treichler, *How to Have Theory in an Epidemic: Cultural Chronicles of AIDS* (Durham, NC: Duke University Press. 1999).

33 Lorraine Daston and Peter Galison, *Objectivity* (Cambridge, MA: MIT Press, 2010).

34 Lianne McTavish, *Childbirth and the Display of Authority in Early Modern France* (Burlington, VT: Ashgate, 2005).

35 Robert Nye, "Medicine and Science as Masculine 'Fields of Honor,'" *Osiris* 12 (1997): 60–79.

36 Steven Shapin, *Leviathan and the Air-Pump: Hobbes, Boyle, and the Experimental Life* (Princeton, NJ: Princeton University Press, 1985).

37 Mario Biagioli, *Galileo, Courtier: The Practice of Science in the Culture of Absolutism* (Chicago: University of Chicago Press, 1993).

38 Kathryn Montgomery, *How Doctors Think: Clinical Judgment and the Practice of Medicine* (New York: Oxford University Press, 2006).

39 Ibid., 29–41.

40 Lisa Keränen, *Scientific Characters: Rhetoric, Politics, and Trust in Breast Cancer Research* (Tuscaloosa: University of Alabama Press, 2010).

Notes to pages 13–36 127

41 Pierre Bourdieu, "The Production of Belief: Contribution to an Economy of Symbolic Goods," *Media, Culture and Society* 2 (1980): 261–93.

Chapter 1: Toward a Theory of Medical Disinterestedness

1 Bourdieu's concept of social capital is markedly different from Robert Putnam's. Putnam focused on the value of social connections for the specific purpose of promoting civic engagement, and thus his concept of social capital has an explicitly positive political purpose. See Bob Edwards and Michael W. Foley, "Civil Society and Social Capital beyond Putnam," *American Behavioral Scientist* 42, 1 (1998): 12. Meanwhile, for Bourdieu, social capital is a neutral concept. It is fundamentally a question of "who do you know?"

2 Pierre Bourdieu, *Practical Reason* (Stanford, CA: Stanford University Press), 47 ff, 85; *Outline of a Theory of Practice*, trans. R. Nice (Cambridge: Cambridge University Press, 1977), 41, 179–81; *Science of Science and Reflexivity*, trans. R. Nice (Chicago: University of Chicago Press, 2004), 52.

3 See Bourdieu, *Outline of a Theory of Practice*, 4–8.

4 Ibid., 171–73.

5 Bourdieu, *Distinction: A Social Critique of the Judgement of Taste*, trans. R. Nice (Cambridge, MA: Harvard University Press, 1984), 291.

6 Bourdieu, *Practical Reason*, 102.

7 Bourdieu, "Social Space and Symbolic Power," *Sociological Theory* 7, 1 (1989): 21.

8 Bourdieu, *Outline of a Theory of Practice*, 180, 196; *Distinction*, 80–82, 282, 310; *Practical Reason*, 42–43.

9 Bourdieu, *Distinction*, 55.

10 Bourdieu, *Practical Reason*, 23–24.

11 Ibid.

12 Ibid., 87.

13 Bourdieu, *Science of Science and Reflexivity*, 53.

14 Ibid., 57.

15 Bourdieu, "The Political Field, the Social Science Field, and the Journalistic Field," in *Bourdieu and the Journalistic Field*, ed. R. Benson and E. Neveu (Cambridge: Polity, 2005).

16 Bourdieu, *Practical Reason*, 116.

17 Ibid., 114.

18 Ibid.

19 Ibid., 116.

20 Ibid., 80.

21 Ibid., 80–81.

Chapter 2: A Brotherhood of Scientific Gentlemen

1 Ronald Hamowy, *Canadian Medicine: A Study in Restricted Entry* (Vancouver: Fraser Institute, 1984), 19.

2 Barbara Tunis, "Medical Education and Medical Licensing in Lower Canada: Demographic Factors, Conflict and Social Change," *Histoire sociale/Social History* 27 (May 1981): 70.

3 Maude E. Abbott, *History of Medicine in the Province of Quebec* (Montreal: McGill University Press, 1931), 31–32.

4 Thompson's remedies involved using various botanicals – such as *Lobelia inflata* (also known as Indian tobacco) and red pepper – and steam baths. He opposed the mineral-based remedies of orthodox medicine. (Paul Starr, *The Social Transformation of American Medicine* (New York: Basic Books, 1983), 51).

5 The support for Thompsonians came from the public, consisting of petitions from various districts and churches, including ministers, to the Legislative Assembly ("Thompsonian Petition to the Legislative Assembly," *British American Journal of Medical and Physical Science* 3, 3 (1847): 80. The *Sherbrooke Gazette*, a local newspaper, irked medical men for writing against a stricter regulation of medical practice. See "Quacks and the 'Sherbrooke Gazette,'" *British American Journal of Medical and Physical Science* 5, 9 (1850): 249; "The Sherbrooke Gazette," *British American Journal of Medical and Physical Science* 5, 10 (1850): 276).

6 Medicine in the twentieth century, particularly the first half of the century, was characterized largely by developments in pharmacology, diagnostics, and other laboratory-based biomedicine. See Julius M. Cruse, "History of Medicine: The Metamorphosis of Scientific Medicine in the Ever-Present Past," *American Journal of the Medical Sciences* 318 (1999): 171–80.

7 R.D. Gidney and W.P.J. Millar, *Professional Gentlemen: The Professions in Nineteenth-Century Ontario* (Toronto: University of Toronto Press, 1994), 53.

8 Elizabeth MacNab, *A Legal History of Health Professions in Ontario* (Toronto: Queens Printer, 1970), 9.

9 Geoffrey Bilson, "Canadian Doctors and the Cholera," in *Medicine in Canadian Society: Historical Perspectives*, ed. S.E.D. Shortt (Montreal/Kingston: McGill-Queen's University Press, 1981), 120.

10 Starr, *Social Transformation of American Medicine*, 41–43; Thomas N. Bonner, *Becoming a Physician: Medical Education in Great Britain, France Germany, and the United States, 1750–1945* (Cary, NC: Oxford University Press, 1996), 150.

11 In Britain, there was an intra-professional conflict among medical men, who were divided along political and scientific lines: conservatives sought to maintain medicine as the practice of an elite class of university-educated men, while reformers pushed to dismantle the hierarchy between medicine and surgery and to steer medical education toward a more clinical and practical direction. Paul Underhill, "Alternative Views of Science in Intra-professional Conflict: General Practitioners and the Medical and Surgical Elite 1815–58," *Journal of Historical Sociology* 5, 3 (1992): 322–50.

12 Tunis, "Medical Education and Medical Licensing," 70.

13 Hamowy, *Canadian Medicine*, 80.

14 Ibid.

15 Charles M. Godfrey has documented this struggle in *Medicine for Ontario: A History* (Belleville, ON: Mika, 1979), 46–58.

16 "Correspondence," Editorial, *British American Journal of Medical and Physical Science* 3, 3 (1847): 81.

17 According to Howell, the heroic theory was so deeply entrenched among physicians that many were reluctant to let go of this basis of treatment even after the introduction of aspects of scientific medicine, such as germ theory. See Howell "Elite Doctors and the Development of Scientific Medicine: The Halifax Medical Establishment and 19th Century Medical Professionalism," in *Health, Disease and Medicine: Essays in Canadian History, Proceedings of the First Hannah Conference on the History of Medicine, McMaster University, June 3–5, 1982*, ed. C.G. Roland (Toronto: Hannah Institute for the History of Medicine, 1984), 110.

18 Starr, *Social Transformation of American Medicine*, 38.

19 Michel Foucault, *The Birth of the Clinic: An Archeology of Medical Perception*, trans. A.M. Sheridan (London: Routledge, 2003), 199.

20 Starr, *The Social Transformation of American Medicine*, 51.

21 Howell relates the story of Dr. Frederick W. Morris of Halifax, who was expelled from the Medical Society for treating smallpox with an Indigenous remedy and then endorsing it in public. Howell, "Elite Doctors," 105.

22 "Debate on the Thompsonian Bill," editorial, *British American Journal of Medical and Physical Science* 5, 1 (1849): 25.

23 As a result of this decision homeopaths and Thompsonians (also called eclectics) had representative seats on the Council of the College of Physicians and Surgeons until 1960. George M. Torrance, "Socio-Historical Overview," in *Health and Canadian Society: Sociological Perspectives*, ed. David Coburn, Carl D'Arcy, and George M. Torrance (Pickering, ON: Fitzhenry and Whiteside, 1987), 12.

24 "Medical Men and the Coming Election," correspondence, *British American Journal of Medical and Physical Science* 7, 8 (1851): 363.

25 "Debate on the Thompsonian Bill," *British American Journal of Medical and Physical Science* 5, 1 (1849): 26.

26 "Medical Politics," editorial, *Upper Canada Journal of Medical, Surgical and Physical Science* 1 (1851): 158–68, reprinted in Hamowy, *Canadian Medicine*, 88.

27 "Homeopathic Conversation," *British American Journal of Medical and Physical Science* 7, 2 (1851): 93.

28 See Liz Curtis, *Nothing but the Same Story: The Roots of Anti-Irish Racism* (London: Information on Ireland, 1984); Mary Hickman, *Religion, Class, and Identity: The State, the Catholic Church, and the Education of the Irish in Britain* (Aldershot, UK: Avebury, 1995).

29 "Debate on the Thompsonian Bill, *British American Journal of Medical and Physical Science* 5, 1 (1849): 26.

30 Ibid., 25.

31   Ibid.
32   Starr, *Social Transformation of American Medicine*, 52–53.
33   Lorraine Daston and Peter Galison, *Objectivity* (Cambridge, MA: MIT Press, 2010), 185.
34   Ibid., 198–205.
35   "The Sherbrooke Gazette," *British American Journal of Medical and Physical Science* 5, 10 (1850): 276.
36   In the Legislative Assembly of the United Province of Canada, Dr. Nelson tried to disgrace Thompsonians and homeopaths by quoting Paracelsus, the "prince of Quacks," a disgraced physician during the Renaissance: "The very down on his bald pate had more knowledge than all the writers; the buckles of his shoes more learning than Galen and Avicenna; and his beard more experience than all the universities" ("Debate on the Thompsonian Bill," *British American Journal of Medical and Physical Science* 5, 1 (1849): 26).
37   The proposed bill to modify medical education "would admit a student to practice without having touched a subject or heard a lecture, except upon clinical medicine and surgery: and *this is the mode in which the profession is to be ameliorated!!* Dr. G. will excuse us from 'joining their united appeal' for any such reform, which savours strongly, to our mind, of demolition" ("'Et Tu, Brute!'" *British American Journal of Medical and Physical Science* 5, 1 (1849): 25).
38   Rainer Baehre, "The Medical Profession in Upper Canada Reconsidered: Politics, Medical Reform, and Law in a Colonial Society," *Canadian Bulletin of Medical History / Bulletin canadien d'histoire de la médecine* 12 (1995): 108.
39   Ibid., 106.
40   William Canniff, *The Medical Profession in Upper Canada, 1783–1850: An Historical Narrative with Original Documents relating to the Profession including Some Brief Biographies* (Toronto: William Briggs, 1894), 15–16.
41   For these reasons, American medical schools were often derogatorily called "proprietary schools," although, as Thomas N. Bonner argues, such for-profit schools also existed in Britain (*Becoming a Physician*, 151).
42   Canniff, *The Medical Profession in Upper Canada*, 53.
43   See ibid., 59–61.
44   Sylvio Leblond describes an incident in 1832 where the Quebec Board of Medicine in Lower Canada refused to grant medical licences to four French candidates who received their medical diplomas at the University of Vermont at Burlington, on the grounds that their three-month education did not meet the board's requirement for five years of study in medicine ("La médecine dans la province de Québec avant 1847," *Les cahier des dix* 35 (1970): 81–84). Canniff documents cases where American-educated candidates were rejected by the medical board in Upper Canada. For example, in July 1836 a candidate "from the United States, educated at the University of Maryland and Pennsylvania" was rejected because he "exhibited a total ignorance of the Latin language, and seemed to be as uninformed of English

grammar" (*The Medical Profession in Upper Canada,* 85). In April 1834 another candidate who "presented [a] certificate of attending a course of lectures at Dartmouth, in New Hampshire, and of his proficiency in the Latin language" was rejected because he was "found to be quite ignorant of Latin grammar and was therefore advised to pursue his studies" (ibid., 78).

45 Paul Underhill, "Alternative Views of Science."

46 See Canniff, *The Medical Profession in Upper Canada,* 51, 56–57.

47 Bonner, *Becoming a Physician,* 150; Starr, *Social Transformation of American Medicine,* 42.

48 Underhill, "Alternative Views of Science," 324.

49 Ibid.

50 See Sylvio Leblond's description of open public examinations for medical candidates, which included an audience consisting of medical men, students, parents of candidates, and the curious public ("La medicine," 82).

51 The range of qualities that were organized around rationality and masculine notions of honour meant that certain groups were automatically excluded from the brotherhood of scientific gentlemen. According to Kenan Malik, Victorian race relations in Britain were organized primarily in terms of stratifications within a racial society rather than between different races, so that class-based identification of the poor as a distinctive race, as a group that "could not be considered as part of a common community but should be regarded as a threat to the integrity of society," became the primary focus for Victorian Britons (Malik, *The Meaning of Race: Race, History, and Culture in Western Society* (New York: New York University Press, 1996), 202). Malik argues that colonial racism in the nineteenth century did not develop until the race-based discourse of class had already been established (ibid., 92–97). Hence, women, men of colour, Jewish men, and Aboriginal healers would not have been perceived as viable players in the struggle for status and dominance among medical men, who considered themselves to be a class-race distinct from these subordinate groups. These groups would have been perceived as having no possibility of occupying a viable position in the field of struggles among medical men and as being outside of the limits of the field proper. It is likely for this reason that the few women physicians and midwives who did practise during the nineteenth century did not factor into the debates about the qualities that befitted a medical man as a gentleman.

52 Robert Nye, "Medicine and Science as Masculine 'Fields of Honor,'" *Osiris* 12 (1997): 60–74.

53 In 1865, a revision of the Medical Act was passed that would establish the General Medical Council of Upper Canada, represented by physicians from both the profession and the medical schools, which oversaw membership and licensing. Through this act, examination of potential candidates fell to the individual medical schools. See Gidney and Millar, *Professional Gentlemen,* 10–11.

54 H.E. MacDermot, *History of the Canadian Medical Association, 1867–1921* (Toronto: Murray Printing, 1935), 13.

55 "The Homeopaths and Eclectics," *British American Journal of Medical and Physical Science* 1 (1868): 230.
56 "The Homeopaths and Eclectics," *British American Journal of Medical and Physical Science* 2 (1869): 27.
57 Nye, "Medicine and Science," 63.
58 "Counter-petition to the Governor General," editorial, *British American Journal of Medical and Physical Science* 3 (1848): 246.
59 "The Doings of the 'Repeal Association,'" editorial, *British American Journal of Medical and Physical Science* 3 (1848): 277.
60 "The Medical Bill, and the School of Medicine of Montreal," editorial, *British American Journal of Medical and Physical Science* 2 (1846): 21.
61 Ibid., 22.
62 Ibid., emphasis in original.
63 Ibid.
64 Editorial, "Correspondence," *British American Journal of Medical and Physical Science* 1 (1846): 335.
65 "Professional Etiquette," editorial, *British American Journal of Medical and Physical Science* 1 (1846): 306.
66 Canadian Medical Association, "Code of Ethics of the Canadian Medical Association," 1868, 8, http://www.archive.org/details/cihm_00948.
67 Percival's *Medical Ethics: Or, a Code of Institutes and Precepts, Adapted to the Professional Conduct of Physicians and Surgeons* (Manchester: S. Russell, 1803) became the foundation of the Code of Ethics of the American Medical Association in 1847 and later the Canadian Medical Association in 1868. See P. Sohl and H.A. Bassford, "Codes of Medical Ethics: Traditional Foundations and Contemporary Practice," *Social Science of Medicine* 22 (1986): 1175–79.
68 W. Fraser, "Queries in Medical Ethics," *British American Journal of Medical and Physical Science* 5 (1849): 155.
69 Ibid.
70 Ibid., 306.
71 "Professional Etiquette," editorial, *British American Journal of Medical and Physical Science* 1 (1846): 306.
72 Canadian Medical Association, "Code of Ethics," 13.
73 Ibid, 10.
74 Ibid, 9.
75 Ibid, 13.
76 Michel Foucault, *Security, Territory, Population: Lectures at the Collège de France, 1977–1978*, ed. M. Senellart, trans. G. Burchell (New York: Palgrave Macmillan, 2007).
77 Foucault, *Birth of the Clinic*, 39–40, and *History of Sexuality*, vol. 1, *An Introduction*, trans. R. Hurley (New York: Vintage Books, 1990), 140–45.
78 "Medical Men and the Coming Election," correspondence, *British American Journal of Medical and Physical Science* 7 (1851): 363.

79 Canniff, *The Medical Profession in Upper Canada*, 64.
80 "Debate on the Thompsonian Bill," *British American Journal of Medical and Physical Science* 5, 1 (1849): 26.
81 "Thompsonian Petitions to the Legislative Assembly," editorial, *British American Journal of Medical and Physical Science* 3 (1847): 80.
82 "The Duties of the Government to Our Profession," editorial, *Dominion Medical Journal* 1 (1868): 49.
83 Geoffrey Bilson, *A Darkened House* (Toronto: University of Toronto Press, 1980), 3, 164–65.
84 Linsey McGoey, "Pharmaceutical Controversies and the Performative Value of Uncertainty," *Science as Culture* 18 (2009): 151–64.
85 "The Public Health," editorial, *British American Journal of Medical and Physical Science* 5 (1849): 52.
86 Ibid., 81.
87 "Thompsonian Petitions to the Legislative Assembly," *British American Journal of Medical and Physical Science* 3 (1847): 26.
88 "The Ministry and the Board of Health," editorial, *British American Journal of Medical and Physical Science* 5 (1850): 303.
89 Ibid.

Chapter 3: Building Bridges, Making Amends

1 C. David Naylor, *Private Practice, Public Payment: Canadian Medicine and the Politics of Health Insurance, 1911–1966* (Montreal/Kingston: McGill-Queen's University Press, 1986), 136.
2 Robin F. Badgley and Samuel Wolfe, *Doctors' Strike: Medical Care and Conflict in Saskatchewan* (New York: Atherton Press, 1967), 22.
3 I use the term "medical profession" to refer to the professional group, as represented by the professional interest groups the Saskatchewan Medical Association and the Canadian Medical Association. I use the term "doctors" when discussing diverse opinions that were expressed at the time. Not all doctors were against the plan proposed by the CCF government. Some actively supported it and others did not participate in the walkout because of ethical obligations toward their patients. The historical work on this subject documents that doctors were under strict discipline to project a unified front against the government, and any dissent with the official position of the Saskatchewan Medical Association and the Saskatchewan College of Physicians and Surgeons was suppressed. Although the official discourse of the medical profession does not represent all, or perhaps even most, views held by individual doctors, this discourse is important for understanding how the group chose to present itself to the public, the state, and the media, and within its own ranks, and how this self-representation by professional medicine changed over time.
4 Badgley and Wolfe, *Doctors' Strike*, 88–92.

5   See "Doctors Outside the Law," editorial, *Globe and Mail*, 4 July 1962, 6; "The Democratic Way," editorial, *Globe and Mail*, 7 July 1962, 6.

6   Gregory P. Marchildon and Klaartje Schirjvers, "Physician Resistance and the Forging of Public Healthcare: A Comparative Analysis of the Doctors' Strikes in Canada and Belgium in the 1960s," *Medical History* 55 (2011): 219.

7   Ibid., 219.

8   See Geoffrey Bilson's discussion of medical services and class in Canadian urban centres during the cholera epidemics of the nineteenth century (*A Darkened House* (Toronto: University of Toronto Press, 1980), 14–15).

9   Bagley and Wolfe, *Doctors' Strike*, 78.

10 Quoted in "Health Education of the Public in Canada," editorial, *Canadian Medical Association Journal* (hereafter *CMAJ*) 85 (1961): 1008.

11 L.R. Rabson, "The People's Health: Whose Responsibility?" *CMAJ* 88 (1963): 198.

12 Harry Baker, "Doctor-Patient Relationship or Doctor-Public Relationship," *CMAJ* 78 (1958): 129.

13 See Badgley and Wolfe, *Doctors' Strike*, 8–10.

14 See C. Stuart Houston, "Saskatchewan's Municipal Doctors a Forerunner of the Medicare System That Developed 50 Years Later," *CMAJ* 151 (1994): 1643.

15 See Naylor, *Private Practice*, 182–83; Badgley and Wolfe, *Doctors' Strike*, 17; Malcolm G. Taylor, *Health Insurance and Canadian Public Policy* (Montreal/Kingston: McGill-Queen's University Press, 2009), 276–78.

16 See Taylor, *Health Insurance*, 70–74; E.A. Tollefson, *Bitter Medicine: The Saskatchewan Medicare Feud* (Saskatoon: Modern Press, 1964), 3.

17 Robin F. Badgley and Samuel Wolfe, "The Doctors' Right to Strike," in *Ethical Issues in Medicine: The Role of the Physician in Today's Society*, ed. E.F. Torrey (Boston: Little, Brown, 1968), 311.

18 "The Hammer and the Heritage," editorial, *CMAJ* 87 (1962): 303.

19 Naylor documents the years of negotiations between the Saskatchewan medical profession and the provincial government. See *Private Practice*, 136–43.

20 A.D. Kelly, "The Saskatchewan Situation: One Man's View," *CMAJ* 87 (1962): 1113.

21 See Naylor, *Private Practice*; Taylor, *Health Insurance*.

22 Malcolm Taylor notes that, of these two private companies, Medical Services Incorporated (MSI) insured 217,000, and Group Medical Services (GMS) insured 91,000 (Taylor, *Health Insurance*, 261).

23 J.W. Reid, "Acceptance of Payments from a Third Party," *CMAJ* 88 (1963): 819.

24 "Unjust Laws Exist," editorial, *CMAJ* 87 (1962): 190.

25 G.K. Higgins, "Universal Health Insurance: A Problem of Minority Rights," *CMAJ* 87 (1962): 1383.

26 See Badgley and Wolfe's quotation from the Declaration of Geneva, which all doctors receive a copy of, which "pledges a doctor 'to consecrate my life to the service of humanity; I will practice my profession with conscience and dignity'" ("Doctors' Right to Strike," 319).

27 Kelly, "The Saskatchewan Situation," 1114.
28 The majority of newspapers in Saskatchewan, including the *Regina Leader-Post* and the *Saskatoon Star-Phoenix*, were owned by the Sifton family, which supported the Liberals, who had lost the provincial election to the CCF. The papers editorialized the debates between the medical profession and the government in favour of the former, framing the health care bill as "'a smoke-screen to divert the electorate's attention' from the CCF's impending transformation into a party dominated by organized labour" (Naylor, *Private Practice*, 184).
29 See Joan Hollobon, "A Prairie Doctor and His Conscience," *Globe and Mail*, 4 July 1962, 7; "UK Medical Journals Oppose MD's Strike," *Globe and Mail*, 13 July 1962, 8; "Group Warns MDs to Yield by Friday," *Globe and Mail*, 5 July 1962, 1; Eddie Keen, "My Patients Come First, Says One Non-striker," *Vancouver Province*, 3 July 1962, 2. For other examples, see Taylor, *Health Insurance*, 307–13.
30 See Taylor, *Health Insurance*, 324, 327–30.
31 Eric M. Meslin, "The Moral Costs of the Ontario Physicians' Strike," *Hastings Center Report* 17, 4 (1987): 11–14.
32 L.F. Koyl, "Have We Missed the Boat?" *CMAJ* 74 (1956): 299.
33 Ibid., 300.
34 Francis T. Hodges, "Public Relations Forum: Medicine's Seven Deadly Sins," *CMAJ* 76 (1957): 660.
35 C.P. Harrison, "Fluoridation," *CMAJ* 81 (1959): 128.
36 "The Social Scientist and the Hospital," editorial, *CMAJ* 72 (1955): 857.
37 G.R.F. Elliot, "Teaching of Preventive Medicine in Canada," *CMAJ* 74 (1956): 457.
38 "Medicine and Morals," editorial, *CMAJ* 81 (1959): 744.
39 "Schoolmasters to the Nation," editorial, *CMAJ* 87 (1962): 1030.
40 Koyl, "Have We Missed the Boat?" 299.
41 V.W.J., "The Family Doctor," *CMAJ* 74 (1956): 480.
42 Alexander Robertson, "The Place of Social Medicine," *CMAJ* 82 (1960): 724.
43 S.E.D. Shortt, "'Before the Age of Miracles': The Rise, Fall and Rebirth of General Practice in Canada, 1890–1940," in *Health, Disease and Medicine: Essays in Canadian History: Proceedings of the First Hannah Conference on the History of Medicine, McMaster University, June 3–5, 1982*, ed. C.G. Roland (Toronto: Hannah Institute for the History of Medicine, 1984), 125.
44 V.W.J., "The Family Doctor," 479.
45 Elliot, "Teaching of Preventive Medicine," 459.
46 Koyl, "Have We Missed the Boat?" 209.
47 John Geyman, *The Corrosion of Medicine: Can the Profession Reclaim Its Moral Legacy?* (Monroe, ME: Common Courage Press, 2008), 51.
48 "Health Education of the Public," editorial, *CMAJ* 77 (1957): 135.
49 Ibid.
50 "The Social Scientist and the Hospital," editorial, *CMAJ* 72 (1955): 857.

51 Alexander Robertson, "A Commentary on Sociology in the Medical School," *CMAJ* 84 (1961): 704.

52 F.W. Hanley, "Ethics, the Doctor and the Social Scientist," *CMAJ* 73 (1955): 849.

53 See H.A. Halpin, M.M. Morales-Suarez-Varela, and J.M. Martin-Moreno, "Chronic Disease Prevention and the New Public Health," *New Public Health* 32, 1 (2010): 121–25; B. Starfield, J. Hyde, J. Gervas, and I. Heath, "The Concept of Prevention: A Good Idea Gone Astray?" *Journal of Epidemiological Community Health* 62 (2008): 580–83.

54 G.J. Millar, "'Skip the Health Lesson, Teacher!' A Commentary on Health Education in Canadian Elementary and Secondary Schools," *CMAJ* 86 (1962): 647.

55 Alondra Nelson, *Body and Soul: The Black Panther Party and the Fight against Medical Discrimination* (Minneapolis: University of Minnesota Press, 2013), 75–114.

56 Dorothy Porter, "How Did Social Medicine Evolve, and Where Is It Heading?" *PLoS Medicine* 3, 10 (2006): 1667–72.

57 Robertson, "The Place of Social Medicine," 724.

58 Ibid., 725.

59 Robertson, "A Commentary on Sociology," 703.

60 Robertson, "The Place of Social Medicine," 724.

61 Robertson, "A Commentary on Sociology," 704.

62 Jacalyn Duffin, *History of Medicine: A Scandalously Short Introduction*, 2nd ed. (Toronto: University of Toronto Press, 2010), 382–84.

63 W. Harding LeRiche, "The Family Physician: A Vanishing Canadian?" *CMAJ* 73 (1955): 572.

64 F. Murray Fraser, "Let's Face the Facts," *CMAJ* 85 (1961): 307

65 V.W.J., "The Family Doctor," 479.

66 Ibid.

67 Max Alexandroff, "The Family Physician, 1955," *CMAJ* 72 (1955): 540.

68 Fraser, "Let's Face the Facts," 306.

69 College of Family Physicians, "College History" (n.d.), para 1–3, http://www.cfpc.ca/CollegeHistory/.

70 Robert F. Purtell, "General Practitioners' Duty as Medical Teachers," *CMAJ* 73 (1955): 750.

71 "Committee on Fellowship," editorial, CMAJ 73 (1955): 232–33.

72 "General Practitioner Research," editorial, *CMAJ* 73(1955): 684–85.

73 Fraser, "Let's Face the Facts," 306.

74 Marvin Wellman, "On the Practice of Medicine," *CMAJ* 79 (1958): 189.

75 See Robert Whitaker, "Anatomy of an Epidemic: Psychiatric Drugs and the Astonishing Rise of Mental Illness in America," *Ethical Human Psychology and Psychiatry* 7, 1 (2005): 23–35.

76 In the aftermath of the Second World War, a heightened demand for psychiatric treatment brought together veterans' and mental health programs and propelled what had been predominately an academic discipline of psychology to embrace

clinical psychiatry as a body of knowledge and practice as well as a professional concern. See Robin L. Cautin, "A Century of Psychotherapy, 1860–1960," in *History of Psychotherapy: Continuity and Change*, 2nd ed., ed. John C. Norcross, Gary R. VandenBos, and Donald K. Freedheim, 3–38 (Washington, DC: American Psychological Association, 2011).

77 See American Psychiatric Association, "*DSM* History," para. 6, http://www.psychiatry.org/practice/dsm/dsm-history-of-the-manual.

78 "The Therapeutic Value of Talk," editorial, *CMAJ* 77 (1957): 888.

79 M. Tyndel, "The Role of the General Practitioner in Psychiatry," *CMAJ* 82 (1960): 324.

80 Wellman, "On the Practice of Medicine," 189.

81 Tyndel, "Role of the General Practioner," 324.

82 It would be difficult to entertain this analysis using a governmentality framework because the adoption of the social by doctors would be interpreted as the integration of the medical profession into the biopolitics of the state. However, using a framework informed by Bourdieu allows an examination of how the pressures of public shaming of and declining public trust in the medical profession created a bump in the road to rapid scientization and specialization and significantly reoriented the direction of medicine to the point of reviving what was seen as an outdated form of medicine – general practice.

83 See L.W. Holmes, "A Code of Cooperation," *CMAJ* 76 (1957): 891.

84 L.W. Holmes, "Public Attitudes towards Doctors, V," *CMAJ* 76 (1957): 144–46.

85 L.W. Holmes, "Ambassadors of Goodwill," *CMAJ* 73 (1955): 683–84; L.W. Holmes, "The Doctor Speaks," *CMAJ* 74 (1956): 396–97.

86 Gordon A. Sinclair, "Why Has the Canadian Medical Association a Public Relations Program?" *CMAJ* 78 (1958): 359–60.

87 Ibid., 360.

88 H.B. Atlee, "CMA Public Relations and the Saskatchewan Affair," letter to the editor, *CMAJ* 87 (1962): 878.

89 For a history of public relations, see Robert L. Heath, Elizabeth L. Toth, and Damion Waymer, eds., *Rhetorical and Critical Approaches to Public Relations*, vol. 2 (New York: Routledge, 2009), particularly Chapter 5, "Perspectives on Public Relations History," by Ron Pearson.

90 Sinclair, "Why Has the Canadian Medical Association a Public Relations Program," 359.

91 For Saussurian semiotic approaches that examine this euphemistic strategy in advertising, see Robert Goldman, *Reading Ads Socially* (New York: Routledge, 1992); Judith Williamson, *Decoding Advertisements: Ideology and Meaning in Advertising* (New York: Mario Boyars, 1978); and Stuart Hall, ed., *Representation: Cultural Representations and Signifying Practices* (Thousand Oaks, CA: Sage, 1997). See also Roland Barthes, "Rhetoric of the Image," in *The Visual Culture Reader*, ed. Nicholas Mirzoeff, 135–38 (New York: Routledge, 2002).

92 For the relationship between advertising and public relations, see Robert Jackall and Janice Hirota, *Image Makers: Advertising, Public Relations and the Ethos of Advocacy* (Chicago: University of Chicago Press, 2000).

93 L.W. Holmes, "The Five W's of Medical Public Relations," *CMAJ* 73 (1955): 484.

94 Sinclair, "Why Has the Canadian Medical Association a Public Relations Program," 359.

95 L.W. Holmes, "Preventive PR," *CMAJ* 76 (1957): 229–30.

96 Ibid., 230.

97 L.W. Holmes, "Doctors and Dollars," *CMAJ* 73 (1955): 982.

98 Ibid.

99 Holmes, "Public Attitudes toward Doctors," 145.

100 Holmes, "The Five W's," 484.

101 "The Doctors' Position," Presentation of the Saskatoon and District Medical Society on CFQC-TV, 1 June 1962, Saskatchewan Council for Archives and Archivists, *Medicare: A People's Issue*, http://scaa.sk.ca/gallery/medicare/en_display.php?ref=en_doc-strike&max=113&dir=doctors-strike&img=99.

102 Sinclair, "Why Has the Canadian Medical Association a Public Relations Program?" 360.

103 M. Etziony, "Medical Ethics: Faith, Fossil or Way of Life?" *CMAJ* 84 (1961): 1196–98.

104 Baker, "Doctor-Patient Relationship," 128.

105 Cappon, "CMA Public Relations and the Saskatchewan Affair," *CMAJ* 87 (1962): 625.

106 Atlee, "CMA Public Relations," 878.

107 Cappon, "CMA Public Relations," 625.

108 Atlee, "CMA Public Relations," 878.

109 Cappon, "CMA Public Relations," 625.

110 A.D. Kelly, "The General Secretary Replies," letter to the editor, *CMAJ* 87 (1962): 626–27.

111 Cappon, "CMA Public Relations," 626.

112 Atlee, "CMA Public Relations," 878.

113 Cappon, "CMA Public Relations," 626.

114 "Medicine and the Mass Media," editorial, *CMAJ* 78 (1958): 786.

115 Canadian Medical Association, "Code of Ethics," 1945, 6, www.royalcollege.ca/rcsite/documents/bioethics/cma-code-ethics-1945.pdf.

116 The CMA's code of ethics of 1928 lumped together personal advertising and public relations: "It is derogatory to the dignity of the profession to resort to public advertisements, or private cards, or handbills inviting the attention of individuals affected by particular diseases, publicly offering advice and medicine to the poor gratis, or promising radical cures; to publish cases and operations in the daily prints, or suffer such publication to be made; to invite laymen to be present at operations, to boast of cures and remedies; to adduce certificates of skill and

success, or to perform any other similar acts" (2–3). Ten years later, this section of the code was revised, and individual advertising was separated from "Communications to the Laity on Medical Subjects" (Canadian Medical Association, "Code of Ethics," 1938, 6, www.royalcollege.ca/rcsite/documents/bioethics/cma-code-ethics-1938.pdf).

117 The CMA's code of ethics of 1945 contained wording from the code of ethics of the British Medical Association that forbade doctors from "[discussions] in the lay press on disputed points of pathology or treatment" and from "taking charge of columns in which answers to correspondents on medical questions are printed" (6). These statements are absent from the 1956 version of the code.

118 William Osler, "Internal Medicine as a Vocation," *Medical News* (New York) 71 (1897): 660.

119 Canadian Medical Association, "Code of Ethics," 1938, 6; 1945, 6.

120 Jeremy Iggers, "Contemporary Ethical Concepts in Historical Context," in his *Good News, Bad News: Journalism Ethics and the Public Interest* (Boulder, CO: Westview Press, 1999), 67.

121 See Patrick Champagne and Dominique Marchetti, "The Contaminated Blood Scandal: Reframing Medical News," in *Bourdieu and the Journalistic Field*, ed. Rodney Benson and Erik Neveu (Malden, MA: Polity Press, 2005), 117–18.

122 Baker, "Doctor-Patient Relationship," 131.

123 L.W. Holmes, "The Doctor and the Press," *CMAJ* 74 (1956): 224.

Chapter 4: The Paradox of Medical Publishing

1 The senior editor of the *Journal of the American Medical Association*, George Lundberg, was fired for publishing an article on American college students' perceptions of oral sex during the period of former president Bill Clinton's impeachment trial. See Janice Hopkins Tanne, "*JAMA*'s Editor Fired over Sex Article," *British Medical Journal* 318 (1999): 213.

2 Jerome Kassirer of the *New England Journal of Medicine* disagreed with the journal publisher's new direction to print other medical publications under the journal's name. See Bruce Japsen, "New England Journal of Medicine Fires Top Editor," *Chicago Tribune*, 27 July 1999, http://articles.chicagotribune.com/1999-07-27/business/9907270059_1_dr-jerome-kassirer-massachusetts-medical-society-consumer-newsletters.

3 Bill Curry, "Interference Alleged at Medical Journal," *Globe and Mail*, 22 February 2006, A14.

4 John Hoey, "Sacking of *CMAJ* Editors Is Deeply Troubling," editorial, *Lancet* 367 (2006): 704.

5 Jerome P. Kassirer, Frank Davidoff, Kathryn O'Hara, and Donald A. Redelmeier, "Editorial Autonomy of *CMAJ*," *CMAJ* 174 (2006): 947.

6 Paul Webster, "Canadian Researchers Respond to *CMAJ* Crisis," *Lancet* 367 (2006): 1134.

7 Miriam Shuchman and Donald A. Redelmeier, "Politics and Independence: The Collapse of the *Canadian Medical Association Journal*," *New England Journal of Medicine* 354 (2006): 1339.

8 Laura Eggertson and Barbara Sibbald, "Privacy Issues Raised over Plan B: Women Asked for Names, Addresses, Sexual History," *CMAJ* 173 (2005): 1435–36.

9 Anne McIlroy, "How a Battle for Editorial Independence Came to Cost So Much," *Globe and Mail*, 1 April 2006, A4.

10 Ibid.

11 Curry, "Interference Alleged," A14.

12 "The Editorial Autonomy of *CMAJ*," editorial, *CMAJ* 174 (2006): 9.

13 Kassirer et al., "Editorial Autonomy of *CMAJ*," 945.

14 Ibid.

15 For example, the news media coverage of the Watergate scandal in 1974 made reporters Carl Bernstein and Bob Woodward into heroes. Scholars in journalism studies point out that their Watergate reportage was highly sensationalized (James Aucoin, *The Evolution of American Investigative Journalism* (Columbia: University of Missouri Press, 2005), 17–18; David L. Protess et al., *The Journalism of Outrage: Investigative Reporting and Agenda Building in America* (New York: Guilford Press, 1991), 50–52), yet their reportage still remains a fixture in the popular image of journalism's virtues to shed light on activities of the powerful elite that undermine the common good (this style and approach to investigative reporting is apparent in such films as *The Insider* (1999), about the tobacco industry, and *Fair Game* (2010), about a journalist who writes about how the Bush administration misled the public to justify the invasion of Iraq).

16 Matthew Kieran, *Media Ethics* (New York: Routledge, 1998), 159.

17 Martin Vogel, "Sacking of *CMAJ* Editors," *Lancet* 367 (2006): 1486.

18 For a history of malpractice in medical research, see Andrew Goliszek, *In the Name of Science: A History of Secret Programs, Medical Research, and Human Experimentation* (New York: St. Martin's Press, 2003).

19 See Adriana Petryna, "Globalizing Human Subject Research," in *Global Pharmaceuticals*, ed. Adriana Petryna, Andrew Lakoff, and Arthur Kleinman, 33–60 (Durham, NC: Duke University Press, 2006).

20 Canadian Institutes of Health Research, Natural Sciences and Engineering Research Council of Canada, and Social Sciences and Humanities Research Council of Canada, *Tri-council Policy Statement: Ethical Conduct for Research Involving Humans* 2010: 37–39, http://www.pre.ethics.gc.ca/pdf/eng/tcps2/TCPS_2_FINAL_Web.pdf.

21 Adriana Petryna, "Ethical Variability: Drug Development and Globalizing Clinical Trials," *American Ethnologist* 32 (2006): 183–97.

22 Laura Stark, *Behind Closed Doors: IRBs and the Making of Ethical Research* (Chicago: University of Chicago Press, 2012), 41–55.

23 Jeremy Iggers, *Good News, Bad News: Journalism Ethics and the Public Interest* (Boulder, CO: Westview Press, 1999), 92–93.

24 Lorraine Daston and Peter Galison, *Objectivity* (Cambridge, MA: MIT Press, 2010).
25 Kassirer et al., "Editorial Autonomy of *CMAJ*," 946.
26 Ibid., 947.
27 "Marijuana: Federal Smoke Clears a Little," editorial, *CMAJ* 164 (2001): 1397.
28 Wayne Kondro and Barbara Sibbald, "Tony Clement Appointed as Canada's New Health Minister," *CMAJ* 174 (2006): 754.
29 "Quebec's Bill 114," editorial, *CMAJ* 167 (2002): 617.
30 Ibid.
31 Dana Hanson, "Questions of Trust," *CMAJ* 167 (2002): 986.
32 "A Letter from *CMAJ*'s Editorial Board to the CMA," *CMAJ* 167 (2002): 1230.
33 McIlroy, "How a Battle for Editorial Independence Came to Cost," A4.
34 "Is Medicine Still a Profession?" editorial, *CMAJ* 174 (2006): 743.
35 "Sacking of *CMAJ* Editors Is Deeply Troubling," 704.
36 G.W. Halpenny, "We Must Build Bridges," *CMAJ* 87 (1962): 183–86.
37 Richard Smith, *Trouble with Medical Journals* (London: Royal Society of Medicine Press, 2006), 33–34.
38 Ibid., 33–36.
39 Ibid., 140.
40 Ibid., 144.
41 Ibid., 145.
42 Alan Brookstone, "Crisis at the *CMAJ*," *British Columbia Medical Journal* 48, 3 (2006): 109.
43 Noni MacDonald is quoted as stating that "the controversy has been fuelled by 'explosive anger'" and that the *CMAJ* was "still getting very high quality stuff coming in" (Paul Webster, "Canadian Researchers Respond to *CMAJ* Crisis," *Lancet* 367, 9517 (2006): 1134).
44 Ibid., 1133.
45 David Spurgeon, "Authors Threaten to Withhold Articles from *CMAJ*," *British Medical Journal* 332, 7545 (2006): 812.
46 Amir Attaran, "Finding True North for the *Canadian Medical Association Journal*," *Lancet* 368 (2006): 1309–11.
47 Ibid., 1310.
48 Robert Steinbrook, "Turning the Page at the *CMAJ*," *New England Journal of Medicine* 355 (2006): 547.
49 Attaran, "Finding True North," 1310.
50 Gaye Tuchman, "Objectivity as Strategic Ritual: An Examination of Newsmen's Notions of Objectivity," *American Journal of Sociology* 77 (1972): 661.
51 Noni MacDonald et al., "Editorial Independence for *CMAJ*: Signposts along the Road," *CMAJ* 175 (2006): 453.
52 Ibid.
53 Creative Commons is a non-profit organization that provides legal infrastructure enabling authors of various intellectual and cultural products to share their work

with others and still retain credit for the initial authorship. According to Creative Commons, this approach is a new way of thinking about the protection of intellectual property in more flexible terms that are still within the legal framework of copyright. See http://www.creativecommons.org/about.

54 James Maskalyk, "Why Open Medicine?" *Open Medicine* 1 (2007): E1.
55 John Hoey, Caralee E. Caplan, Tom Elmslie, Kenneth M. Flegel, et al., "Science, Sex and Semantics: The Firing of George Lundberg," *CMAJ* 160 (1999): 508.
56 "Open Access in Medical Publishing: Trends and Countertrends," editorial, *CMAJ* 172 (2005): 149.
57 Smith, *Trouble with Medical Journals*, 151.
58 Ibid.
59 Ibid.
60 "Editorial Policies," *Open Medicine: A Peer-Reviewed, Independent, Open-Access Journal.* http://www.openmedicine.ca/about/editorialpolicies.
61 Ibid.
62 Daston and Galison, *Objectivity*, 312–14.
63 Jerome P. Kassirer, "A Canadian Purge," *BMJ Opinion*, 4 March 2016, https://blogs.bmj.com/bmj/2016/03/04/jerome-p-kassirer-a-canadian-purge/.
64 Canadian Press, "Canadian Medical Journal, *Open Medicine*, Stops Publishing," *Canadian Broadcasting Corporation News*, 4 November 2014, https://www.cbc.ca/news/health/canadian-medical-journal-open-medicine-stops-publishing-1.2823643.
65 Marco Chown Oved, "Canadian Medical Journals Hijacked for Junk Science," *Toronto Star*, 29 September 2016.

Conclusion

1 In 2016 at a spring conference of Canadian Association of Nurses in AIDS Care (CANAC), M.T. O'Shaughnessy made the point, when considering health care and the roles one plays in it, that, at some point, all individuals – whether physician, nurse, radiologist, and so on – are eventually in the role of patient.

Selected Bibliography

Abbott, Maude E. *History of Medicine in the Province of Quebec*. Montreal: McGill University Press, 1931.

Armstrong, David. "Embodiment and Ethics: Constructing Medicine's Two Bodies." *Sociology of Health and Illness* 28, 6 (2006): 866–81. https://doi.org/10.1111/j.1467-9566.2006.00547.x.

Armstrong, David, and Jane Ogden. "The Role of Etiquette and Experimentation in Explaining How Doctors Change Behavior: A Qualitative Study." *Sociology of Health and Illness* 28, 7 (2006): 951–68. https://doi.org/10.1111/j.1467-9566.2006.00514.x.

Aucoin, James L. *The Evolution of American Investigative Journalism*. Columbia: University of Missouri Press, 2005.

Badgley, Robin F., and Samuel Wolfe. "The Doctors' Right to Strike." In *Ethical Issues in Medicine: The Role of the Physician in Today's Society*, ed. E.F. Torrey, 301–21. Boston: Little, Brown, 1968.

–. *Doctors' Strike: Medical Care and Conflict in Saskatchewan*. New York: Atherton Press, 1967.

Baehre, Rainer. "The Medical Profession in Upper Canada Reconsidered: Politics, Medical Reform, and Law in a Colonial Society." *Canadian Bulletin of Medical History / Bulletin canadien d'histoire de la médecine* 12 (1995): 101–24. https://doi.org/10.3138/cbmh.12.1.101.

Balsamo, Anne. *Technologies of the Gendered Body: Reading Cyborg Women*. Durham, NC: Duke University Press, 1996.

Barthes, Roland. "Rhetoric of the Image." In *The Visual Culture Reader*, ed. Nicholas Mirzoeff, 135–38. New York: Routledge, 2002.

Becker, Howard S., Blanche Geer, Everett C. Hughes, and Anselm L. Strauss. *Boys in White: Student Culture in Medical School*. New Brunswick, NJ: Transaction, 1977.

Benson, R., and E. Neveu, eds. *Bourdieu and the Journalistic Field*. Cambridge: Polity, 2005.

Berg, Marc, and Annmarie Mol, eds. *Differences in Medicine: Unravelling Practices, Techniques and Bodies*. Durham, NC: Duke University Press, 1998.

Biagioli, Mario. *Galileo, Courtier: The Practice of Science in the Culture of Absolutism*. Chicago: University of Chicago Press, 1993.

Bilson, Geoffrey. "Canadian Doctors and the Cholera." In *Medicine in Canadian Society: Historical Perspectives*, ed. S.E.D. Shortt, 115–36. Montreal/Kingston: McGill-Queen's University Press, 1981.

–. *A Darkened House*. Toronto: University of Toronto Press, 1980.

Bonner, Thomas N. *Becoming a Physician: Medical Education in Great Britain, France, Germany, and the United States, 1750–1945*. Cary, NC: Oxford University Press, 1996.

Bourdieu, Pierre. *Distinction: A Social Critique of the Judgement of Taste*, trans. R. Nice. Cambridge, MA: Harvard University Press, 1984.

–. *Outline of a Theory of Practice*, trans. R. Nice. Cambridge: Cambridge University Press, 1977.

–. "The Political Field, the Social Science Field, and the Journalistic Field." In *Bourdieu and the Journalistic Field*, ed. R. Benson and E. Neveu, 29–47. Cambridge: Polity, 2005.

–. *Practical Reason*. Stanford, CA: Stanford University Press, 1998.

–. "The Production of Belief: Contribution to an Economy of Symbolic Goods." *Media, Culture and Society* 2 (1980): 261–93. https://doi.org/10.1177/016344378000200305.

–. *Science of Science and Reflexivity*, trans. R. Nice. Chicago: University of Chicago Press, 2004.

–. "Social Space and Symbolic Power." *Sociological Theory* 7, 1 (1989): 14–25. https://doi.org/10.2307/202060.

Britten, Nicky. "Prescribing and the Defense of Clinical Autonomy." *Sociology of Health and Illness* 23, 4 (2001): 478–96. https://doi.org/10.1111/1467-9566.00261.

Brookstone, Alan. "Crisis at the CMAJ." *British Columbia Medical Journal* 48, 3 (2006): 109.

Canadian Institutes of Health Research, Natural Sciences and Engineering Research Council of Canada, and Social Sciences and Humanities Research Council of Canada. *Tri-council Policy Statement: Ethical Conduct for Research Involving Humans*, 2010. http://www.pre.ethics.gc.ca/pdf/eng/tcps2/TCPS_2_FINAL_Web.pdf.

Canniff, William. *The Medical Profession in Upper Canada 1783–1850: An Historical Narrative with Original Documents relating to the Profession, including Some Brief Biographies*. Toronto: William Briggs, 1894.

Cartwright, Lisa. *Screening the Body: Tracing Medicine's Visual Culture*. Minneapolis: University of Minnesota Press, 1995.

Cautin, Robin L. "A Century of Psychotherapy, 1860–1960." In *History of Psychotherapy: Continuity and Change*, 2nd ed., ed. John C. Norcross, Gary R. VandenBos, and Donald K. Freedheim, 3–38. Washington, DC: American Psychological Association, 2011.

Champagne, Patrick, and Dominique Marchetti. "The Contaminated Blood Scandal: Reframing Medical News." In *Bourdieu and the Journalistic Field*, ed. Rodney Benson and Erik Neveu, 113–34. Malden, MA: Polity Press, 2005.

Clarke, Adele, and Virginia Olsen. *Revisioning Women, Health and Healing: Feminist, Cultural and Technoscience Perspectives*. New York: Routledge, 1999.

Coburn, David. "Canadian Medicine: Dominance or Proletarianization?" *Milbank Quarterly* 66, Suppl. 2 (1988): 92–116. https://doi.org/10.2307/3349917.

–. "State Authority, Medical Dominance, and Trends in the Regulation of the Health Professions: The Ontario Case." *Social Science and Medicine* 37, 2 (1993): 129–38. https://doi.org/10.1016/0277-9536(93)90137-S.

Coburn, David, George M. Torrance, and Joseph M. Kaufert. "Medical Dominance in Canada in Historical Perspective: The Rise and Fall of Medicine?" *International Journal of Health Services* 13, 3 (1983): 407–32. https://doi.org/10.2190/D94Q-0F9Y-VYQH-PX2V.

Cruse, Julius M. "History of Medicine: The Metamorphosis of Scientific Medicine in the Ever-Present Past." *American Journal of the Medical Sciences* 318 (1999): 171–80. https://doi.org/10.1016/S0002-9629(15)40609-3.

Curtis, Liz. *Nothing but the Same Story: The Roots of Anti-Irish Racism*. London: Information on Ireland, 1984.

Daston, Lorraine, and Peter Galison. *Objectivity*. Cambridge, MA: MIT Press, 2010.

Duffin, Jaclyn. *History of Medicine: A Scandalously Short Introduction*. 2nd ed. Toronto: University of Toronto Press, 2010.

Duster, Troy. *Backdoor to Eugenics*. New York: Routledge, 2003.

Edwards, Bob, and Michael W. Foley. "Civil Society and Social Capital beyond Putnam." *American Behavioral Scientist* 42, 1 (1998): 12. https://doi.org/10.1177/0002764298042001010.

Foucault, Michel. *The Birth of Biopolitics: Lectures at the Collège de France 1978–1979*, ed. M. Senellart, trans. G. Burchell. New York: Palgrave Macmillan, 2008.

–. *The Birth of the Clinic: An Archeology of Medical Perception*, trans. A.M. Sheridan. London: Routledge, 2003.

–. *The History of Sexuality*. Vol. 1, *An Introduction*, trans. R. Hurley. New York: Vintage Books, 1990.

–. *Madness and Civilization: A History of Insanity in the Age of Reason*, trans. R. Howard. New York: Vintage, 1988.

–. *Security, Territory, Population: Lectures at the Collège de France, 1977–1978*, ed. M. Senellart, trans. G. Burchell. New York: Palgrave, 2007.

Fraser, Suzanne, and kylie valentine. *Substance and Substitution: Methadone Subjects in Liberal Societies*. New York/Basingstoke, UK: Palgrave Macmillan, 2008.

Friedson, E. *Profession of Medicine: A Study of the Sociology of Applied Knowledge*. Chicago: University of Chicago Press, 1970.

Geyman, John. *The Corrosion of Medicine: Can the Profession Reclaim Its Moral Legacy?* Monroe, ME: Common Courage Press, 2008.

Gidney, R.D., and W.P.J. Millar. "The Origins of Organized Medicine in Ontario, 1850–1869." In *Health, Disease and Medicine: Essays in Canadian History. Proceedings of the First Hannah Conference on the History of Medicine, McMaster University, June 3–5, 1982*, ed. C.G. Roland, 65–95. Toronto: Hannah Institute for the History of Medicine, 1984.

–. *Professional Gentlemen: The Professions in Nineteenth-Century Ontario*. Toronto: University of Toronto Press, 1994.

Gilman, Sander L. "AIDS and Syphilis: The Iconography of Disease." In *AIDS: Cultural Analysis/Cultural Activism*, ed. Douglas Crimp, 87–107. Cambridge, MA: October Books, 1988. https://doi.org/10.2307/3397566.

Godfrey, Charles M. *Medicine for Ontario: A History*. Belleville, ON: Mika, 1979.

Goldman, Robert. *Reading Ads Socially*. New York: Routledge, 1992.

Goliszek, Andrew. *In the Name of Science: A History of Secret Programs, Medical Research, and Human Experimentation*. New York: St. Martin's Press, 2003.

Grover, Jan Zita. "AIDS: Keywords." In *AIDS: Cultural Analysis/Cultural Activism*, ed. Douglas Crimp, 17–30. Cambridge, MA: October Books, 1988. https://doi.org/10.2307/3397563.

Hacking, Ian. *The Social Construction of What?* Cambridge, MA: Harvard University Press, 1999.

Hall, Stuart., ed. *Representation: Cultural Representations and Signifying Practices*. Thousand Oaks, CA: Sage, 1997.

Halpin, H.A., M.M. Morales-Suarez-Varela, and J.M. Martin-Moreno. "Chronic Disease Prevention and the New Public Health." *New Public Health* 32, 1 (2010): 120–54.

Hammonds, Evelyn. "Towards a Geneology of Black Female Sexuality: The Problematic Silence." In *Feminist Theory and the Body: A Reader*, ed. Janet Price and Margaret Shildrick, 245–59. New York: Routledge, 1997.

Hamowy, Ronald. *Canadian Medicine: A Study in Restricted Entry*. Vancouver: Fraser Institute, 1984.

Heath, Robert L., Elizabeth L. Toth, and Damion Waymer, eds. *Rhetorical and Critical Approaches to Public Relations*. Vol. 2. New York: Routledge, 2009.

Hickman, Mary. *Religion, Class, and Identity: The State, the Catholic Church, and the Education of the Irish in Britain*. Aldershot, UK: Avebury, 1995.

Hightower, Renady. "Ethnography of the Habitus of the Emergency Physician." PhD diss., Wayne State University, 2010.

Holloway, K.J. "Teaching Conflict: Professionalism and Medical Education." *Journal of Bioethical Inquiry* 12, 4 (2015): 675–85.

Howell, Colin D. "Elite Doctors and the Development of Scientific Medicine: The Halifax Medical Establishment and 19th Century Medical Professionalism." In *Health, Disease and Medicine: Essays in Canadian History: Proceedings of the First*

Hannah Conference on the History of Medicine, McMaster University, June 3–5, 1982, ed. C.G. Roland, 105–22. Toronto: Hannah Institute for the History of Medicine, 1984.

Iggers, Jeremy. *Good News, Bad News: Journalism Ethics and the Public Interest.* Boulder, CO: Westview Press, 1999.

Institute of Medicine. *Conflict of Interest in Medical Research, Education, and Practice.* Washington, DC: National Academies Press, 2009.

Jackall, Robert, and Janice Hirota. *Image Makers: Advertising, Public Relations and the Ethos of Advocacy.* Chicago: University of Chicago Press, 2000.

Keränen, Lisa. *Scientific Characters: Rhetoric, Politics, and Trust in Breast Cancer Research.* Tuscaloosa: University of Alabama Press, 2010.

Kieran, Matthew. *Media Ethics.* New York: Routledge, 1998.

King, Samantha. *Pink Ribbon, Inc.: Breast Cancer and the Politics of Philanthropy.* Minneapolis: University of Minnesota Press, 2006.

Latour, Bruno. *Pasteurization of France,* trans. A. Sheridan and J. Law. Cambridge, MA: Harvard University Press, 1988.

Leblond, Sylvio. "La médecine dans la province de Québec avant 1847." *Les cahiers des dix* 35 (1970): 65–95. https://doi.org/10.7202/1025271ar.

Lexchin, Joel. "Those Who Have the Gold Make the Evidence: How the Pharmaceutical Industry Biases the Outcomes of Clinical Trials of Medications." *Science and Engineering Ethics* 18, 2 (2012): 247–61. https://doi.org/10.1007/s11948-011-9265-3.

Luke, Haida. *Medical Education and Sociology of Medical Habitus: "It's Not about the Stethoscope!"* Boston: Kluwer Academic, 2003.

MacDermot, H.E. *History of the Canadian Medical Association, 1867–1921.* Toronto: Murray Printing, 1935.

MacNab, Elizabeth. *A Legal History of Health Professions in Ontario.* Toronto: Queen's Printer, 1970.

Malik, Kenan. *The Meaning of Race: Race, History, and Culture in Western Society.* New York: New York University Press, 1996.

Marchildon, Gregory P., and Klaartje Schirjvers. "Physician Resistance and the Forging of Public Healthcare: A Comparative Analysis of the Doctors' Strikes in Canada and Belgium in the 1960s." *Medical History* 55, 2 (2011): 203–22.

McGoey, Linsey. "Pharmaceutical Controversies and the Performative Value of Uncertainty." *Science as Culture* 18 (2009): 151–64. https://doi.org/10.1080/09505430902885474.

McKinlay, John, and Joan Arches. "Towards the Proletarianization of Physicians." *International Journal of Health Services* 15 (1985): 161–95. https://doi.org/10.2190/JBMN-C0W6-9WFQ-Q5A6.

McTavish, Lianne. *Childbirth and the Display of Authority in Early Modern France.* Burlington, VT: Ashgate, 2005.

Meslin, Eric M. "The Moral Costs of the Ontario Physicians' Strike." *Hastings Center Report* 17, 4 (1987): 11–14.

Mol, Annmarie. *The Logic of Care: Health Care and the Problem of Choice*. Abingdon, UK/New York: Routledge, 2008.

Montgomery, Kathryn. *How Doctors Think: Clinical Judgment and the Practice of Medicine*. New York: Oxford University Press, 2006. ProQuest Ebook Central. http://lib.myilibrary.com?ID=53312.

Navarro, Vicente. "Professional Dominance or Proletarianization? Neither." *Milbank Quarterly* 66, Suppl. 2 (1988): 57–75. https://doi.org/10.2307/3349915.

Naylor, C. David. *Private Practice, Public Payment: Canadian Medicine and the Politics of Health Insurance, 1911–1966*. Montreal/Kingston: McGill-Queen's University Press, 1986.

Neatby, Hilda. "The Medical Profession in the North-West Territories." In *Medicine in Canadian Society: Historical Perspectives*, ed. S.E.D. Shortt, 165–88. Montreal/Kingston: McGill-Queen's University Press, 1981.

Nelson, Alondra. *Body and Soul: The Black Panther Party and the Fight against Medical Discrimination*. Minneapolis: University of Minnesota Press, 2013.

Nettleton, Sarah, Roger Burrows, and Ian Watt. "Regulating Medical Bodies? The Consequences of the 'Modernisation' of the NHS and the Disembodiment of Clinical Knowledge." *Sociology of Health and Illness* 30, 3 (2008): 333–48. https://doi.org/10.1111/j.1467-9566.2007.01057.x.

Nye, Robert. "Medicine and Science as Masculine 'Fields of Honor." *Osiris* 12 (1997): 60–79. https://doi.org/10.1086/649267.

Oldani, Michael. "Thick Prescriptions: Toward an Interpretation of Pharmaceutical Sales Practices. *Medical Anthropology Quarterly* 18, 3 (2004): 325–56. https://doi.org/10.1525/maq.2004.18.3.325.

Osborne, Thomas. "Medicine and Epistemology: Michel Foucault and the Liberality of Clinical Reason." *History of the Human Sciences* 5, 2 (1992): 63–93. https://doi.org/10.1177/095269519200500204.

Patton, Cindy. *Inventing AIDS*. New York: Routledge, 1990.

–. *Rebirth of the Clinic*. Minneapolis: University of Minnesota Press, 2010.

–. *Sex and Germs: The Politics of AIDS*. Boston: South End Press, 1985.

Patton, Cindy, and John Liesch. "In Your Face." In *Cosmetic Surgery: A Feminist Primer*, ed. Cressida J. Hayes and Meredith Jones, 209–24. Farnham, UK/Burlington, VT: Ashgate, 2009.

Percival, Thomas. *Medical Ethics: Or, a Code of Institutes and Precepts, Adapted to the Professional Conduct of Physicians and Surgeons*. Manchester: S. Russell, 1803.

Petryna, Adriana. "Ethical Variability: Drug Development and Globalizing Clinical Trials." *American Ethnologist* 32 (2006): 183–97. https://doi.org/10.1525/ae.2005.32.2.183.

–. "Globalizing Human Subject Research." In *Global Pharmaceuticals*, ed. Adriana Petryna, Andrew Lakoff, and Arthur Kleinman, 33–60. Durham, NC: Duke University Press, 2006.

Petryna, Adriana, Andrew Lakoff, and Arthur Kleinman, eds. *Global Pharmaceuticals*. Durham, NC: Duke University Press, 2006.

Porter, Dorothy. "How Did Social Medicine Evolve and Where Is It Heading?" *PLOS Medicine* 3, 10 (2006): 1667–72. https://doi.org/10.1371/journal.pmed.0030399.

Protess, David L., Fay Lomax Cook, Jack C. Doppelt, James S. Ettema, Margaret T. Gordon, Donna R. Leff, and Peter Miller. *The Journalism of Outrage: Investigative Reporting and Agenda Building in America.* New York: Guilford Press, 1991.

Rose, Nikolas. *The Politics of Life Itself: Biomedicine, Power and Subjectivity in the Twenty-First Century.* Princeton, NJ: Princeton University Press, 2007.

Ruhl, P. Lealle. "Liberal Governance and Prenatal Care." *Economy and Society* 28 (1999): 95–117. https://doi.org/10.1080/03085149900000026.

Shapin, Steven. *Leviathan and the Air-Pump: Hobbes, Boyle, and the Experimental Life.* Princeton, NJ: Princeton University Press, 1985.

Shortt, S.E.D. "Antiquarians and Amateurs: Reflections on the Writing of Medical History." In *Medicine in Canadian Society: Historical Perspectives,* ed. S.E.D. Shortt, 1–18. Montreal/Kingston: McGill-Queen's University Press, 1981.

–. "'Before the Age of Miracles': The Rise, Fall and Rebirth of General Practice in Canada, 1890–1940." In *Health, Disease and Medicine: Essays in Canadian History: Proceedings of the First Hannah Conference on the History of Medicine, McMaster University, June 3–5, 1982,* ed. C.G. Roland, 123–52. Toronto: Hannah Institute for the History of Medicine, 1984.

–. "Physicians, Science, and Status: Issues in the Professionalization of Anglo-American Medicine in the Nineteeth Century." *Medical History* 27 (1983): 51–68. https://doi.org/10.1017/S0025727300042265.

Sismondo, Sergio. "Ghosts in the Machine: Publication Planning in the Medical Sciences." *Social Studies of Science* 39, 2 (2009): 171–98. https://doi.org/10.1177/0306312708101047.

Smith, Richard. *Trouble with Medical Journals.* London: Royal Society of Medicine Press, 2006.

Sohl, P., and H.A. Bassford. "Codes of Medical Ethics: Traditional Foundations and Contemporary Practice." *Social Science of Medicine* 22 (1986): 1175–79.

Sontag, Susan. *AIDS and Its Metaphors.* New York: Farrar, Straus and Giroux, 1989.

Starfield, B., J. Hyde, J. Gervas, and I. Heath. "The Concept of Prevention: A Good Idea Gone Astray?" *Journal of Epidemiological Community Health* 62 (2008): 580–83. https://doi.org/10.1136/jech.2007.071027.

Stark, Laura. *Behind Closed Doors: IRBs and the Making of Ethical Research.* Chicago: University of Chicago Press, 2012.

Starr, Paul. *The Social Transformation of American Medicine.* New York: Basic Books, 1983.

Stone, Deborah A. "The Doctor as Businessman: The Changing Politics of a Cultural Icon." *Journal of Health Politics, Policy and Law* 22, 2 (1997): 533–56. https://doi.org/10.1215/03616878-22-2-533.

Strong-Boag, Veronica. "Canada's Women Doctors: Feminism Constrained." In *Medicine in Canadian Society: Historical Perspectives*, ed. S.E.D. Shortt, 207–36. Montreal/Kingston: McGill-Queen's University Press, 1981.

Taylor, Malcolm G. *Health Insurance and Canadian Public Policy*. Montreal/Kingston: McGill-Queen's University Press, 2009.

Thorne, Sally E., Susan R. Harris, Karen Mahoney, Andrea Con, and Liza McGuinness. "The Context of Health Care Communication in Chronic Illness." *Patient Education and Counseling* 54 (2004): 299–306. https://doi.org/10.1016/j.pec.2003.11.009.

Tollefson, E.A. *Bitter Medicine: The Saskatchewan Medicare Feud*. Saskatoon: Modern Press, 1964.

Torrance, George M. "Socio-Historical Overview." In *Health and Canadian Society: Sociological Perspectives*, ed. David Coburn, Carl D'Arcy, and George M. Torrance, 6–32. Pickering, ON: Fitzhenry and Whiteside, 1987.

Treichler, Paula A. *How to Have Theory in an Epidemic: Cultural Chronicles of AIDS*. Durham, NC: Duke University Press, 1999.

Treichler, Paula, Lisa Cartwright, and Constance Penley. *The Visible Woman: Imaging Technologies, Gender, and Science*. New York: New York University Press, 1998.

Tuchman, Gaye. "Objectivity as Strategic Ritual: An Examination of Newsmen's Notions of Objectivity." *American Journal of Sociology* 77 (1972): 660–79. https://doi.org/10.1086/225193.

Tunis, Barbara. "Medical Education and Medical Licensing in Lower Canada: Demographic Factors, Conflict and Social Change." *Histoire sociale/Social History* 27 (May 1981): 67–91.

–. "Medical Licensing in Lower Canada: The Disputes over Canada's First Medical Degree." In *Medicine in Canadian Society: Historical Perspectives*, ed. S.E.D. Shortt, 137–64. Montreal/Kingston: McGill-Queen's University Press, 1981.

Underhill, Paul. "Alternative Views of Science in Intra-professional Conflict: General Practioners and the Medical and Surgical Elite 1815–58." *Journal of Historical Sociology*, 5, 3 (1992): 322–50. https://doi.org/10.1111/j.1467-6443.1992.tb00029.x.

Weir, Lorna. *Pregnancy, Risk and Biopolitics: On the Threshold of the Living Subject*. London: Routledge, 2006.

Wendell, Susan. *Rejected Body: Feminist Philosophical Reflections on Disability*. New York: Routledge, 1996.

West, Candace. "When the Doctor Is a 'Lady': Power, Status and Gender in Physician-Patient Encounters." *Symbolic Interaction* 7, 1 (1984): 87–106. https://doi.org/10.1525/si.1984.7.1.87.

Whitaker, Robert. "Anatomy of an Epidemic: Psychatric Drugs and the Astonishing Rise of Mental Illness in America." *Ethical Human Psychology and Psychiatry* 7, 1 (2005): 23–35. https://doi.org/10.3109/01612840.2012.713447.

William, A.P., E. Vayda, M.L. Cohen, C.A. Woodward, and B.M. Ferrier. "Medicine and the Canadian State: From the Politics of Conflict to the Politics of

Accommodation?" *Journal of Health and Social Behavior* 36, 4 (1995): 303–21. https://doi.org/10.2307/2137321.

Williamson, Judith. *Decoding Advertisements: Ideology and Meaning in Advertising.* New York: Mario Boyars, 1978.

Willis, Evan. "Introduction: Taking Stock of Medical Dominance." *Health Sociological Review* 15 (2006): 421–31. https://doi.org/10.5172/hesr.2006.15.5.421.

Index

advertising, 89. *See also* public relations and media work
anatomy, 41, 47–48
anti-economic universes, 13, 14, 22, 25, 32
Armstrong, David, 9–10
Attaran, Amir, 113
autonomous and heteronomous spaces, 26–28
autonomy, editorial, 98, 106, 108–9, 110–11, 114–16, 117

Badgley, Robin F., 72
behavioural models, 80, 81, 82–83, 86
Biagioli, Mario, 12
biopolitics, 60, 73
Bourdieu, Pierre: on anti-economic universes, 13, 14, 22; approach to, 15, 18–19; on autonomous and heteronomous spaces in journalism, 26; on balancing intellectual capital and bureaucratic principle in science, 25–26; on bourgeoisie, 23; on euphemisms, 31; field theory, 19, 22–23; on gift giving, 20, 32, 63–64; on habitus and double habitus, 9, 19, 28–30, 32; revival of general medicine and, 137n82; on symbolic capital, 20–21. *See also* medical (invested) disinterestedness
bourgeoisie, 22, 23–24, 27, 50–51, 54
British American Journal of Medical and Physical Science, 40, 43–44, 53–54, 56–57
British Medical Journal (BMJ), 110
brotherhood, 55–56
bureaucratic principle, 25–26, 27

Canadian Medical Association (CMA): code of ethics on public relations, 92–93, 138n116, 139n117; original code of ethics, 50, 55–56, 57, 58–59; reframing public relations for doctors, 87–90
Canadian Medical Association Journal (CMAJ): on contrast between medicine and journalism, 94; on incorporation of the social, 78–79,